Introduction

Welcome to ***"The Diverticulitis Cookbook: 110+ Delicious and Soothing Recipes."*** This book is crafted with care and expertise to serve as a comprehensive guide for those navigating the challenges of diverticulitis, a condition that affects the digestive system and requires mindful eating to manage symptoms and promote healing.

Diverticulitis, a common gastrointestinal disorder, involves the inflammation or infection of small pouches (diverticula) that can form in the walls of the colon. Managing this condition often means making significant adjustments to your diet, focusing on foods that reduce inflammation and provide soothing relief. This cookbook aims to transform these dietary adjustments from a daunting task into a delightful culinary journey.

Inside these pages, you will discover over 110 carefully curated recipes designed to be both delicious and gentle on the digestive system. Whether you're experiencing an acute flare-up or maintaining a balanced diet to prevent future episodes, you'll find a wide variety of recipes to suit your needs. From hearty breakfasts and satisfying lunches to comforting dinners and indulgent desserts, this collection ensures that every meal is a pleasure, not a chore.

Each recipe is developed with specific ingredients that are known to be beneficial for diverticulitis sufferers. You'll find tips on how to incorporate fiber gradually into your diet, understand which foods to avoid, and learn cooking techniques that enhance digestibility and nutrient absorption. The recipes are straightforward, using readily available ingredients and easy-to-follow instructions, making them accessible even for those who might be new to cooking.

In addition to recipes, this cookbook includes a comprehensive introduction to understanding diverticulitis, its symptoms, and the importance of dietary choices in managing the condition. You'll also find meal planning advice, shopping lists, and tips for dining out, empowering you to take control of your health through informed food choices.

"The Diverticulitis Cookbook" is more than just a collection of recipes; it's a supportive companion on your journey to better health. By embracing these delicious and soothing dishes, you can alleviate discomfort, enhance your well-being, and rediscover the joy of eating.

Embark on this culinary adventure and let the healing power of food guide you towards a healthier, happier life.

1. Overnight oats with chia seeds and berries

Ingredients:
- 1/2 cup old-fashioned rolled oats
- 1/2 cup milk of your choice (dairy, almond, oat, etc.)
- 1/4 cup plain Greek yogurt
- 1 tbsp chia seeds
- 1 tbsp maple syrup or honey
- 1/2 tsp vanilla extract
- 1/2 cup fresh or frozen berries (strawberries, blueberries, raspberries, etc.)

Instructions:

1. In a jar or bowl with a lid, combine the oats, milk, yogurt, chia seeds, maple syrup/honey, and vanilla. Stir well to combine.

2. Cover and refrigerate overnight or for at least 6 hours to allow the oats to soften and absorb the liquid.

3. In the morning, remove from the fridge and stir well. The chia seeds should have expanded into a gel-like consistency.

4. Fold in the fresh or frozen berries.

5. Serve chilled and enjoy! You can top with extra berries, nuts, coconut, etc. if desired.

Notes:
- This makes 1 single serving, so multiply ingredients as needed.

- For thicker oats, use less milk. For thinner, use more milk to your desired consistency.

- Can use any yogurt you prefer - plain, vanilla, etc. Greek yogurt adds protein.

The overnight oats and chia provide a filling, fiber-rich breakfast with the fresh berries adding natural sweetness and antioxidants. It's a healthy and delicious make-ahead breakfast option!

2. Avocado toast on whole wheat bread

Ingredients:
- 2 slices whole wheat bread
- 1 ripe avocado
- 1 tbsp lemon or lime juice
- 1/4 tsp salt
- 1/4 tsp black pepper
- 1 tsp olive oil or avocado oil (optional)
- Toppings of your choice (examples: red pepper flakes, everything bagel seasoning, feta cheese, cherry tomatoes, sprouts, etc.)

Instructions:
1. Toast the two slices of whole wheat bread until lightly browned and crunchy.

2. Cut the avocado in half, remove the pit, and scoop the flesh into a small bowl. Add the lemon/lime juice, salt, and pepper.

3. Use a fork to mash the avocado until it reaches your desired consistency (some prefer it chunky, others smooth).

4. Optional: Drizzle the olive oil or avocado oil over the mashed avocado and stir to incorporate.

5. Divide the mashed avocado between the two toasted bread slices, spreading it evenly over the surface.

6. Add any desired toppings over the avocado toast. Some delicious options include:
   - Red pepper flakes
   - Everything bagel seasoning
   - Crumbled feta or goat cheese
   - Sliced cherry tomatoes
   - Sprouts or microgreens, Drizzle of balsamic glaze

7. Serve the avocado toast immediately while the bread is warm and toasty.

Notes:
- For added protein, you can put a fried or poached egg on top.
- Swap whole wheat for multigrain, sourdough or rye bread if desired.
- Sprinkle with sesame seeds, chia seeds or hemp hearts for extra nutrition.

Avocado toast makes a filling, healthy and delicious breakfast or snack with good fats, fiber and nutrients from the whole grains and avocado.

3. Yogurt parfait with granola and fruit

Ingredients:
- 1 cup plain Greek yogurt or yogurt of your choice
- 1/2 cup granola
- 1 cup fresh fruit (berries, bananas, mango, etc.), diced
- 2 tbsp honey or maple syrup (optional)
- 1 tsp vanilla extract (optional)
- Cinnamon or other spices to taste (optional)

Instructions:

1. In a bowl or parfait glass, layer 1/4 of the yogurt on the bottom.

2. Top with 1/4 of the granola and 1/4 of the fresh diced fruit.

3. Drizzle with a little honey or maple syrup if you want it sweetened. You can also add a dash of vanilla and/or cinnamon at this layer.

4. Repeat the layers once more: yogurt, granola, fruit, optional sweeteners/spices.

5. For the final top layer, add the remaining yogurt and granola.

6. If desired, you can add some extra fruit, nuts, coconut, etc. as a garnish on top.

7. Refrigerate for 30 minutes to 1 hour before serving to allow flavors to meld if possible.

8. Serve chilled and enjoy! The granola will soften slightly from the yogurt.

Notes:
- Get creative with different yogurt flavors like vanilla, honey, etc.
- Use any fresh fruits you enjoy - mixed berries, tropical fruits, etc.
- Can use low-fat or non-fat yogurts if preferred.
- For extra protein, use Greek yogurt or add nut butters.

This yogurt parfait is not only delicious but provides protein, fiber, vitamins and minerals from the yogurt, fruit and granola. It makes a great breakfast, snack or dessert!

4. Egg white omelet with spinach and mushrooms

Ingredients:
- 1 cup egg whites (around 8 egg whites)
- 1 tsp olive oil or cooking spray
- 1/2 cup sliced mushrooms
- 1 cup fresh baby spinach
- 2 tbsp feta or goat cheese (optional)
- Salt and pepper to taste

Instructions:

1. Crack the eggs and separate the whites from the yolks over a bowl, reserving 1 cup of egg whites.

2. Heat a small nonstick skillet over medium heat and add the olive oil or cooking spray.

3. Add the sliced mushrooms and cook for 2-3 minutes until starting to brown.

4. Add the fresh spinach and cook for 1 more minute until wilted. Season with a pinch of salt and pepper.

5. Pour in the egg whites and let them spread out to coat the pan evenly. Use a spatula to gently push the cooked edges towards the center as it cooks.

6. When the bottom is set but the top is still a bit runny, sprinkle on the feta or goat cheese if using.

7. Use the spatula to fold one side of the omelet over onto itself to form a half-moon shape.

8. Slide the folded omelet onto a plate and season with additional salt and pepper if desired.

9. Serve the egg white omelet warm, optionally with whole grain toast or a side of fruit.

Notes:
- For extra protein, you can add 1-2 egg whites or egg whites.
- Other veggie additions could include tomatoes, onions, bell peppers etc.
- Use any cheese you prefer or omit for a dairy-free version.
- For more flavor, add dried herbs, hot sauce, salsa, etc.

This high protein, veggie-packed egg white omelet makes a nutritious and tasty breakfast option that is low in calories but high in vitamins and minerals.

5. Smoothie with almond milk, banana, and peanut butter

Ingredients:
- 1 cup unsweetened almond milk
- 1 ripe banana
- 2 tbsp peanut butter
- 1 tbsp honey or maple syrup (optional)
- 1 tsp vanilla extract (optional)
- 1/2 cup ice cubes

Instructions:

1. Add the almond milk, banana, peanut butter, honey/maple syrup (if using), and vanilla extract (if using) to a blender.

2. Add the ice cubes to the blender.

3. Blend on high speed until smooth and creamy, about 1 minute.

4. If it's too thick, add a splash more almond milk. If too thin, add a few more ice cubes.

5. Once blended to your desired consistency, pour into a glass.

6. Optional toppings: sprinkle with cinnamon, cocoa powder, granola, extra banana slices or peanut butter on top.

7. Serve immediately while cold and enjoy with a spoon or straw!

Notes:
- For extra protein, you can add a scoop of protein powder.

- Substitute any other nut butter like almond or cashew butter.

- Use frozen banana chunks instead of fresh for an extra thick smoothie.

- Can use any other milk like oat, coconut, dairy etc.

- Add spinach or kale for extra nutrients.

This creamy, protein-packed smoothie is sweet, nutty and so satisfying. It makes a great on-the-go breakfast or snack loaded with fiber, healthy fats and nutrients.

6. Lentil soup

Ingredients:
- 1 cup dried green or brown lentils, rinsed
- 1 tbsp olive oil
- 1 onion, diced
- 2 carrots, diced
- 2 celery stalks, diced
- 3 cloves garlic, minced
- 1 tsp ground cumin
- 1⁄4 tsp dried thyme
- 6 cups vegetable or chicken broth
- 1 bay leaf
- 2 cups chopped kale or spinach (optional)
- 2 tbsp lemon juice
- Salt and pepper to taste

Instructions:

1. In a large pot, heat the olive oil over medium heat. Add the diced onions, carrots and celery. Cook for 5 minutes until softened.

2. Add the minced garlic, cumin and thyme. Cook for 1 minute until fragrant.

3. Add the rinsed lentils, broth and bay leaf. Increase heat to high and bring to a boil.

4. Once boiling, reduce heat to low, cover and simmer for 20-25 minutes, until lentils are tender.

5. Remove bay leaf. Use an immersion blender to partially blend the soup if you prefer a thicker texture (or leave fully brothy).

6. Stir in the chopped greens (kale or spinach) if using and the lemon juice.

7. Season to taste with salt and pepper.

8. Let simmer for 5 more minutes to allow flavors to meld.

9. Serve the lentil soup warm, optionally with crusty bread on the side.

Notes:
- For a richer soup, use chicken broth instead of vegetable broth.
- Can add diced tomatoes, carrots or other vegetables.
- A parmesan rind simmered in the broth adds great flavor.
- Top with fresh parsley, croutons, olive oil or pesto for extra flavor.

This lentil soup is budget-friendly, nutritious and so comforting. It's loaded with plant-based protein and fiber from the lentils.

7. Baked sweet potato with black beans and salsa

Ingredients:
- 4 medium sweet potatoes
- 1 (15oz) can black beans, drained and rinsed
- 1 cup salsa (your preferred type)
- ¼ cup chopped cilantro or green onions
- 1 tbsp olive oil or avocado oil
- 1 tsp ground cumin
- Salt and pepper to taste
- Toppings: avocado, Greek yogurt or sour cream, cheese, etc. (optional)

Instructions:
1. Preheat oven to 400°F. Line a baking sheet with foil or parchment paper.

2. Use a fork to prick holes all over the sweet potatoes. Place them on the prepared baking sheet.

3. Rub the sweet potatoes all over with the olive oil and season with salt and pepper.

4. Bake for 45-60 minutes, until a knife inserted in the thickest part goes in easily. Cooking time will vary depending on size.

5. While the sweet potatoes bake, prepare the black bean topping. In a saucepan, combine the drained black beans, salsa, cumin and chopped cilantro/green onions.

6. Heat the black bean mixture, stirring occasionally, until it's warmed through.

7. Once sweet potatoes are done, slice lengthwise and open them up to create a well in the middle.

8. Scoop some of the warm black bean salsa mixture into each sweet potato well. Top with desired toppings like avocado, sour cream/yogurt, cheese, etc. Serve the loaded sweet potatoes while warm.

Notes:
- Feel free to add in spices, garlic, jalapeno to the black bean mixture.
- Use your favorite salsa variety - fresh, smoky, spicy, etc.
- For extra protein, top with cooked ground turkey or chicken.
- Sweet potatoes can be microwaved if short on time.

This makes a delicious, satisfying vegetarian meal with protein from the beans, vitamin A from sweet potatoes and lots of flavor!

8. Quinoa vegetable stir-fry

Ingredients:
- 1 cup uncooked quinoa, rinsed
- 2 cups vegetable or chicken broth
- 2 tbsp sesame oil or vegetable oil
- 1 red bell pepper, sliced
- 1 cup broccoli florets
- 1 cup snow peas or sugar snap peas
- 1 cup shredded cabbage or coleslaw mix
- 3 cloves garlic, minced
- 2 tsp freshly grated ginger (or 1 tsp ground ginger)
- 2 tbsp low-sodium soy sauce
- 1 tbsp rice vinegar
- 1 tsp sesame seeds
- 2 green onions, sliced
- Salt and pepper to taste

Instructions:
1. Cook the quinoa according to package instructions, using the veggie or chicken broth instead of water.

2. In a large skillet or wok, heat the sesame or vegetable oil over medium-high heat.

3. Add the sliced bell pepper, broccoli, snow peas and cabbage. Stir-fry for 3-4 minutes.

4. Add the minced garlic and grated ginger. Stir-fry for 1 more minute until fragrant.

5. Add the soy sauce and rice vinegar to the vegetable mixture and toss to coat.

6. Add the cooked quinoa and sesame seeds. Gently toss everything together until well combined.

7. Remove from heat and stir in the sliced green onions. Season with salt and pepper to taste. Serve the quinoa veggie stir-fry immediately, while hot.

Notes:
- Feel free to add other veggies like mushrooms, carrots, bean sprouts etc.
- For extra protein, add baked tofu, edamame, chicken or shrimp.
- Swap tamari or coconut aminos for the soy sauce to make gluten-free.
- Top with crushed peanuts or cashews for added crunch.

This quinoa veggie stir-fry is nutrient-packed, high in protein and fiber, and full of fresh flavors. It makes a healthy, satisfying vegetarian meal.

9. Grilled salmon with roasted asparagus

Ingredients:
- 4 (6oz) salmon fillets
- 2 tbsp olive oil, divided
- 1 lb asparagus, tough ends trimmed
- 1 lemon, sliced into wedges
- Salt and pepper to taste
- Dried dill or other herbs like thyme (optional)

For the Salmon:
1. Brush the salmon fillets lightly with 1 tbsp of the olive oil on both sides. Season with salt, pepper and dried dill if desired.

2. Prepare a grill for direct high-heat cooking.

3. Grill the salmon fillets for 4-5 minutes per side until cooked through and opaque in the center. The fish should flake easily with a fork.

For the Asparagus:
1. Preheat oven to 400°F.

2. Trim the woody bottom ends off the asparagus spears.

3. On a baking sheet, toss the asparagus with the remaining 1 tbsp olive oil and season with salt and pepper. Roast for 12-15 minutes, shaking the pan halfway, until spears are crisp-tender.

To Serve:
1. Transfer the grilled salmon fillets to plates.

2. Arrange the roasted asparagus spears alongside the salmon. Garnish with lemon wedges to squeeze over the fish and veggies.

Notes:
- For added flavor, grill lemon slices alongside salmon for squeezing over top.
- Brush salmon with a glaze like teriyaki, pesto or garlic-herb before grilling if desired.
- Bake the salmon instead of grilling if preferred at 400°F for 12-15 minutes.
- You can sub broccolini or green beans for the asparagus.

This is a light, nutritious meal with lean protein from the salmon and fiber from the roasted asparagus. It's easy, flavorful and perfect for spring/summer.

10. Turkey chili with brown rice

Ingredients:
- 1 tbsp olive oil
- 1 onion, diced
- 3 cloves garlic, minced
- 1 lb ground turkey
- 2 tbsp chili powder
- 2 tsp cumin
- 1 tsp dried oregano
- 1/4 tsp cayenne pepper (optional for heat)
- 1 (28oz) can diced tomatoes
- 1 (15oz) can kidney beans, drained and rinsed
- 1 (15oz) can black beans, drained and rinsed
- 1 cup low-sodium chicken or vegetable broth
- Salt and pepper to taste
- Chopped green onions/cilantro for garnish
- 1 cup cooked brown rice, for serving

Instructions:
1. In a large pot, heat the olive oil over medium-high heat. Add the diced onion and cook for 2-3 minutes until translucent.

2. Add the garlic and ground turkey. Cook while crumbling the turkey until browned, about 5 minutes.

3. Stir in the chili powder, cumin, oregano, cayenne (if using), and a pinch each of salt and pepper.

4. Pour in the diced tomatoes with their juices, the kidney beans, black beans and broth.

5. Bring the chili to a simmer. Reduce heat to medium-low and let it simmer for 15-20 minutes, stirring occasionally, to allow flavors to meld.

6. Taste and adjust seasoning as needed, adding more salt/pepper if desired.

7. While the chili simmers, cook the brown rice according to package instructions. Serve the turkey chili over bowls of the cooked brown rice. Garnish with chopped green onions and cilantro.

Notes:
- For a thicker chili, use less broth or mash some beans.
- Add corn, bell peppers or other favorite chili ingredients.
- Top with cheese, avocado, sour cream or crushed tortilla chips.
- Use ground chicken or beef instead of turkey if desired.
- Let it simmer for 30+ minutes for even more developed flavor.

This hearty, protein-packed turkey chili served over fiber-rich brown rice makes for a nourishing and satisfying meal!

11. Vegetable lasagna with whole wheat noodles

Ingredients:

Lasagna:
- 9 whole wheat lasagna noodles
- 2 tbsp olive oil
- 1 onion, diced
- 3 cloves garlic, minced
- 2 cups sliced mushrooms
- 1 red bell pepper, diced
- 1 zucchini, diced
- 1 eggplant, diced
- 1 (28 oz) can diced tomatoes

- 2 tsp dried basil
- 1 tsp dried oregano
- 1/2 tsp salt
- 1/4 tsp black pepper

Cheese Filling:
- 15 oz ricotta cheese
- 1 cup shredded mozzarella cheese
- 1/2 cup grated Parmesan cheese
- 1 egg
- 2 tbsp chopped fresh parsley

Instructions:

1. Preheat oven to 375°F (190°C).

2. Bring a large pot of salted water to a boil. Cook the whole wheat lasagna noodles according to package instructions until al dente. Drain and set aside.

3. In a large skillet, heat the olive oil over medium heat. Add the onion and garlic and sauté for 2-3 minutes until fragrant.

4. Add the mushrooms, bell pepper, zucchini, and eggplant. Cook for 5-7 minutes, stirring occasionally, until the vegetables are tender.

5. Stir in the diced tomatoes, basil, oregano, salt, and pepper. Simmer for 10 minutes, allowing the flavors to meld.

6. In a medium bowl, mix together the ricotta, mozzarella, Parmesan, egg, and parsley for the cheese filling.

7. Spread 1 cup of the vegetable mixture in the bottom of a 9x13 inch baking dish. Arrange 3 lasagna noodles over the top. Spread half of the cheese filling over the noodles, then top with another 1 cup of the vegetable mixture.

8. Repeat the layers of noodles, cheese filling, and vegetables. Top with the remaining 3 noodles and the remaining vegetable mixture.

9. Cover the dish with aluminum foil and bake for 30 minutes. Remove the foil and bake for an additional 15-20 minutes, until the top is bubbly and lightly browned. Let the lasagna cool for 10-15 minutes before slicing and serving.

12. Chicken fajitas with bell peppers and onions

Ingredients:
- 1 lb boneless, skinless chicken breasts, sliced into thin strips
- 2 tbsp olive oil
- 1 tbsp chili powder
- 1 tsp cumin
- 1 tsp garlic powder
- 1/2 tsp smoked paprika
- 1/2 tsp salt
- 1/4 tsp black pepper
- 1 red bell pepper, sliced into thin strips
- 1 green bell pepper, sliced into thin strips
- 1 yellow onion, sliced into thin strips
- 8-10 small whole wheat tortillas or fajita-size flour tortillas
- Toppings (optional): guacamole, salsa, sour cream, shredded cheese

Instructions:
1. In a large bowl, combine the chicken strips, 1 tbsp olive oil, chili powder, cumin, garlic powder, smoked paprika, salt, and pepper. Toss to coat the chicken evenly.

2. Heat the remaining 1 tbsp of olive oil in a large skillet or cast-iron pan over high heat.

3. Add the seasoned chicken to the hot pan and cook for 5-7 minutes, stirring occasionally, until the chicken is cooked through and lightly browned.

4. Remove the chicken from the pan and set aside.

5. In the same pan, add the sliced bell peppers and onions. Sauté for 5-7 minutes, until the vegetables are tender-crisp.

6. Return the cooked chicken to the pan with the vegetables. Stir to combine and heat through.

7. Serve the chicken fajita mixture warm, with the whole wheat or flour tortillas and desired toppings such as guacamole, salsa, sour cream, and shredded cheese.

Tips:
- Adjust the spices to your desired level of heat and flavor.
- For extra juiciness, add a squeeze of fresh lime juice to the chicken and vegetables.
- Serve the fajitas with a side of cilantro-lime rice or black beans.
- Leftovers can be stored in the refrigerator for 3-4 days and reheated in the microwave or on the stovetop.

13. Tuna salad stuffed avocado

Ingredients:
- 2 (5 oz) cans of tuna, drained
- 2 tbsp mayonnaise
- 1 tbsp Dijon mustard
- 1 tbsp lemon juice
- 2 tbsp finely diced celery
- 2 tbsp finely diced red onion
- 2 tbsp chopped fresh parsley
- 1/4 tsp salt
- 1/8 tsp black pepper
- 2 ripe avocados, halved and pitted

Instructions:

1. In a medium bowl, combine the drained tuna, mayonnaise, Dijon mustard, lemon juice, celery, red onion, parsley, salt, and pepper. Mix well until the tuna salad is evenly seasoned.

2. Carefully scoop out the flesh from the avocado halves, leaving about 1/4 inch of avocado flesh attached to the skin to create a "boat" for the tuna salad.

3. Chop the scooped-out avocado flesh and gently fold it into the tuna salad mixture.

4. Spoon the tuna salad mixture evenly into the avocado boats, piling it up slightly in the center.

5. Serve the tuna salad stuffed avocados immediately, or refrigerate until ready to serve.

Tips:
- For extra crunch, add diced cucumber, bell pepper, or toasted almonds to the tuna salad.

- Sprinkle the stuffed avocados with a bit of paprika or cayenne pepper for a touch of heat.

- Serve the stuffed avocados on a bed of mixed greens or with whole grain crackers for a complete meal.

- Use canned wild-caught tuna for a more sustainable and nutritious option.

- Adjust the amount of mayonnaise to your desired creaminess.

Enjoy this healthy and satisfying tuna salad stuffed avocado!

14. Veggie and hummus wrap in a whole wheat tortilla

Ingredients:
- 4 whole wheat tortillas or wraps
- 1 cup hummus (store-bought or homemade)
- 1 cup shredded carrots
- 1 cup thinly sliced cucumber
- 1 cup baby spinach or arugula
- 1/2 cup thinly sliced red bell pepper
- 1/4 cup thinly sliced red onion
- 2 tbsp crumbled feta cheese (optional)
- Salt and pepper to taste

Instructions:

1. Lay the whole wheat tortillas or wraps on a clean surface.

2. Spread about 1/4 cup of hummus evenly over the center of each tortilla, leaving a 1-inch border.

3. Arrange the shredded carrots, sliced cucumber, spinach/arugula, bell pepper, and red onion in a line down the center of each tortilla, on top of the hummus.

4. If using, sprinkle the crumbled feta cheese over the vegetables.

5. Season with a pinch of salt and pepper.

6. Fold the bottom of the tortilla up over the filling, then fold in the sides and continue rolling the tortilla tightly into a wrap.

7. Slice the wrap in half diagonally, if desired, and serve immediately.

Tips:
- Use your favorite variety of hummus, such as classic, roasted red pepper, or garlic.
- Customize the vegetables based on your preferences - try adding avocado, sprouts, or sun-dried tomatoes.
- For extra protein, add grilled or roasted chicken, chickpeas, or tofu.
- Wrap the prepared wraps in parchment paper or foil to enjoy on the go.
- Store any leftover wraps in the refrigerator for up to 3 days.

Enjoy this healthy and flavorful veggie and hummus wrap!

15. Baked cod with roasted Brussels sprouts

Ingredients:

Cod:
- 4 (6 oz) cod fillets
- 2 tbsp olive oil
- 1 tsp lemon zest
- 1 tbsp lemon juice
- 1 tsp Dijon mustard
- 1 tsp dried parsley
- 1/2 tsp salt
- 1/4 tsp black pepper

Brussels Sprouts:
- 1 lb Brussels sprouts, trimmed and halved
- 2 tbsp olive oil
- 1 tsp garlic powder
- 1/2 tsp salt
- 1/4 tsp black pepper

Instructions:

1. Preheat your oven to 400°F (200°C).

2. In a small bowl, whisk together the 2 tbsp olive oil, lemon zest, lemon juice, Dijon mustard, dried parsley, salt, and pepper. Set aside.

3. Arrange the cod fillets in a baking dish and brush or spoon the lemon-herb mixture over the top, making sure to coat the fish evenly.

4. In a separate large bowl, toss the trimmed and halved Brussels sprouts with the 2 tbsp olive oil, garlic powder, salt, and pepper until well coated.

5. Spread the seasoned Brussels sprouts in a single layer on a large baking sheet.

6. Place the baking dish with the cod and the baking sheet with the Brussels sprouts in the preheated oven.

7. Bake for 15-18 minutes, or until the cod is opaque and flakes easily with a fork, and the Brussels sprouts are tender and lightly browned. Serve the baked cod immediately, with the roasted Brussels sprouts on the side.

Tips:
- For extra flavor, add lemon wedges, chopped parsley, or a drizzle of lemon-garlic butter to the cod.
- Roast the Brussels sprouts for a few extra minutes if you prefer them more crispy.
- Try other types of firm white fish, such as halibut or tilapia, in place of the cod.
- Serve the cod and Brussels sprouts with a side of quinoa, roasted potatoes, or a fresh salad for a complete meal.

16. Chickpea curry over brown rice

Ingredients:

Chickpea Curry:
- 2 tbsp olive oil
- 1 onion, diced
- 3 cloves garlic, minced
- 1 tbsp grated fresh ginger
- 2 tsp garam masala
- 1 tsp ground cumin
- 1 tsp ground coriander
- 1/2 tsp ground turmeric
- 1 cup coconut milk
- 1/4 tsp cayenne pepper (or to taste)
- 1 (15 oz) can chickpeas, drained and rinsed
- 1 (14 oz) can diced tomatoes
- 1 tsp salt
- 1/4 cup chopped fresh cilantro

Brown Rice:
- 1 cup uncooked brown rice
- 2 cups water or low-sodium vegetable broth
- 1/4 tsp salt

Instructions:

1. Cook the brown rice: In a medium saucepan, combine the brown rice, water or broth, and 1/4 tsp salt. Bring to a boil, then reduce heat to low, cover, and simmer for 25-30 minutes, until the rice is tender. Fluff with a fork.

2. Make the chickpea curry: In a large skillet or Dutch oven, heat the olive oil over medium heat. Add the diced onion and sauté for 5 minutes until translucent.

3. Add the minced garlic and grated ginger to the pan and cook for 1 minute, until fragrant.

4. Stir in the garam masala, cumin, coriander, turmeric, and cayenne pepper. Cook for 2 minutes to toast the spices.

5. Add the drained and rinsed chickpeas, diced tomatoes, coconut milk, and 1 tsp salt. Bring the mixture to a simmer and cook for 10-15 minutes, stirring occasionally, until the sauce has thickened.

6. Remove from heat and stir in the chopped fresh cilantro. To serve, spoon the chickpea curry over the cooked brown rice.

Tips:
- Adjust the amount of cayenne pepper to control the level of heat. For a creamier curry, use full-fat coconut milk.

- Serve with naan bread, mango chutney, or a fresh green salad on the side. Leftovers can be stored in the refrigerator for 3-4 days or frozen for up to 3 months.

Enjoy this flavorful and nutritious chickpea curry over wholesome brown rice!

17. Turkey burger with roasted sweet potato fries

Ingredients:
Turkey Burgers:
- 1 lb ground turkey
- 1/4 cup breadcrumbs
- 1 egg, lightly beaten
- 2 tbsp finely chopped onion
- 1 tsp Dijon mustard
- 1 tsp Worcestershire sauce
- 1/2 tsp garlic powder
- 1/2 tsp salt
- 1/4 tsp black pepper
- 4 whole wheat burger buns

Sweet Potato Fries:
- 2 lbs sweet potatoes, peeled and cut into 1/2-inch thick fries
- 2 tbsp olive oil
- 1 tsp paprika
- 1/2 tsp garlic powder
- 1/2 tsp salt
- 1/4 tsp black pepper

Instructions:
Sweet Potato Fries:
1. Preheat oven to 400°F (200°C). Line a large baking sheet with parchment paper.
2. In a large bowl, toss the sweet potato fries with the olive oil, paprika, garlic powder, salt, and pepper until evenly coated.
3. Spread the fries in a single layer on the prepared baking sheet.
4. Bake for 20-25 minutes, flipping halfway, until the fries are tender and lightly browned.

Turkey Burgers:
1. In a large bowl, combine the ground turkey, breadcrumbs, egg, onion, Dijon mustard, Worcestershire sauce, garlic powder, salt, and pepper. Mix gently until just combined.
2. Divide the turkey mixture into 4 equal portions and shape them into patties, about 4-5 inches wide and 1/2 inch thick.
3. Heat a large skillet or grill pan over medium-high heat. Cook the turkey burgers for 4-5 minutes per side, or until they reach an internal temperature of 165°F (75°C).
4. Serve the turkey burgers on the whole wheat buns, topped with your favorite condiments.

Assemble: Place a turkey burger on each bun and serve with the roasted sweet potato fries on the side.

Tips:
- For extra flavor, add cheese, avocado, or sautéed mushrooms to the turkey burgers.
- Bake the sweet potato fries in batches if they don't fit in a single layer on the baking sheet.
- Experiment with different seasonings for the sweet potato fries, such as chili powder or cumin.
- Leftovers can be stored in the refrigerator for 3-4 days and reheated in the oven or air fryer.

18. Shrimp stir-fry over quinoa

Ingredients:
- 1 pound shrimp, peeled and deveined
- 2 cups cooked quinoa
- 1 bell pepper, sliced
- 1 onion, sliced
- 2 cloves garlic, minced
- 1 cup broccoli florets
- 1 carrot, julienned
- 2 tablespoons soy sauce
- 1 tablespoon sesame oil
- 1 tablespoon olive oil
- 1 teaspoon ginger, grated
- Salt and pepper to taste
- Optional garnishes: sesame seeds, chopped green onions

Instructions:
1. Heat olive oil in a large skillet or wok over medium-high heat.

2. Add the sliced onion and bell pepper to the skillet and cook for 2-3 minutes until they start to soften.

3. Add the minced garlic and grated ginger to the skillet and cook for another minute until fragrant.

4. Add the shrimp to the skillet and cook for 2-3 minutes until they turn pink and opaque.

5. Stir in the broccoli florets and julienned carrot, and cook for an additional 2-3 minutes until the vegetables are tender-crisp.

6. In a small bowl, mix together the soy sauce and sesame oil.

7. Pour the sauce over the shrimp and vegetable mixture in the skillet and toss to coat everything evenly. Cook for another minute to heat through.

8. Taste and adjust seasoning with salt and pepper if needed.

9. To serve, spoon the cooked quinoa onto plates or bowls, and top with the shrimp stir-fry mixture.

10. Garnish with sesame seeds and chopped green onions if desired.

19. Lentil and vegetable soup

Ingredients:
- 1 cup dry lentils, rinsed and drained
- 4 cups vegetable broth
- 1 onion, diced
- 2 carrots, diced
- 2 celery stalks, diced
- 2 cloves garlic, minced
- 1 can (14 oz) diced tomatoes
- 1 teaspoon dried thyme
- 1 teaspoon dried oregano
- 1 bay leaf
- Salt and pepper to taste
- 2 cups chopped spinach or kale
- 2 tablespoons olive oil
- Optional garnish: chopped fresh parsley, lemon wedges

Instructions:
1. In a large pot, heat the olive oil over medium heat. Add the diced onion, carrots, and celery. Cook for about 5 minutes until the vegetables are softened.

2. Add the minced garlic to the pot and cook for another minute until fragrant.

3. Stir in the rinsed lentils, diced tomatoes (with their juices), dried thyme, dried oregano, bay leaf, and vegetable broth. Bring the mixture to a boil.

4. Once boiling, reduce the heat to low and let the soup simmer for about 20-25 minutes, or until the lentils are tender.

5. Stir in the chopped spinach or kale and cook for an additional 5 minutes until the greens are wilted.

6. Taste the soup and season with salt and pepper according to your preference. Remove the bay leaf.

7. If you prefer a smoother consistency, you can use an immersion blender to partially blend the soup, leaving some chunks of vegetables and lentils intact.

8. Serve the lentil and vegetable soup hot, garnished with chopped fresh parsley and lemon wedges if desired.

20. Grilled portobello mushroom caps stuffed with quinoa

Ingredients:
- 4 large portobello mushroom caps
- 1 cup cooked quinoa
- 1/2 cup diced bell pepper (any color)
- 1/4 cup diced red onion
- 2 cloves garlic, minced
- 1/2 cup diced tomatoes
- 1/4 cup chopped fresh parsley
- 1/4 cup crumbled feta cheese (optional)
- 2 tablespoons olive oil
- 1 tablespoon balsamic vinegar
- Salt and pepper to taste
- Cooking spray

Instructions:
1. Preheat your grill to medium-high heat.

2. Clean the portobello mushroom caps by gently wiping them with a damp paper towel to remove any dirt. Remove the stems and gills from the mushroom caps using a spoon, being careful not to break the caps.

3. In a bowl, mix together the cooked quinoa, diced bell pepper, diced red onion, minced garlic, diced tomatoes, chopped parsley, and crumbled feta cheese (if using). Season with salt and pepper to taste.

4. In a separate small bowl, whisk together the olive oil and balsamic vinegar.

5. Brush the outside of the mushroom caps with the olive oil and balsamic vinegar mixture. Season with salt and pepper.

6. Spoon the quinoa mixture into each mushroom cap, pressing gently to pack it in.

7. Lightly spray the grill grates with cooking spray to prevent sticking. Place the stuffed mushroom caps on the grill, stuffed side up.

8. Grill the mushroom caps for about 8-10 minutes, or until the mushrooms are tender and the filling is heated through.

9. Carefully remove the stuffed mushroom caps from the grill using tongs.

10. Serve the grilled portobello mushroom caps stuffed with quinoa immediately, garnished with additional chopped parsley if desired.

21. Bean and vegetable burritos on whole wheat tortillas

Ingredients:
- 4 whole wheat tortillas
- 1 can (15 oz) black beans, drained and rinsed
- 1 cup cooked brown rice
- 1 bell pepper, diced
- 1 onion, diced
- 1 cup corn kernels (fresh, frozen, or canned)
- 1 cup diced tomatoes
- 1 teaspoon chili powder
- 1/2 teaspoon ground cumin
- 1/2 teaspoon smoked paprika
- Salt and pepper to taste
- 1 cup shredded cheese (cheddar, Monterey Jack, or Mexican blend)
- Optional toppings: diced avocado, salsa, Greek yogurt or sour cream, chopped cilantro

Instructions:

1. Preheat your oven to 350°F (175°C).

2. In a large skillet, heat a bit of oil over medium heat. Add the diced onion and bell pepper. Cook for 3-4 minutes until softened.

3. Add the corn kernels, diced tomatoes, chili powder, ground cumin, smoked paprika, salt, and pepper to the skillet. Cook for another 2-3 minutes, stirring occasionally.

4. Add the black beans and cooked brown rice to the skillet. Stir to combine and cook for another 2-3 minutes until heated through. Taste and adjust seasoning if needed.

5. Place a portion of the bean and vegetable mixture onto each whole wheat tortilla, leaving a border around the edges. Sprinkle shredded cheese over the filling.

6. Fold the sides of each tortilla over the filling, then roll up tightly from the bottom to enclose the filling.

7. Place the rolled burritos seam-side down on a baking sheet lined with parchment paper or aluminum foil.

8. Bake the burritos in the preheated oven for 10-15 minutes, or until the tortillas are lightly crisp and the cheese is melted.

9. Remove the baked burritos from the oven and let them cool slightly before serving.

10. Serve the bean and vegetable burritos on whole wheat tortillas with your favorite toppings such as diced avocado, salsa, Greek yogurt or sour cream, and chopped cilantro.

22. Chicken and veggie stew over brown rice

Ingredients:
- 4 whole wheat tortillas
- 1 can (15 oz) black beans, drained and rinsed
- 1 cup cooked brown rice
- 1 bell pepper, diced
- 1 onion, diced
- 1 cup corn kernels (fresh, frozen, or canned)
- 1 cup diced tomatoes
- 1 teaspoon chili powder
- 1/2 teaspoon ground cumin
- 1/2 teaspoon smoked paprika
- Salt and pepper to taste
- 1 cup shredded cheese (cheddar, Monterey Jack, or Mexican blend)
- Optional toppings: diced avocado, salsa, Greek yogurt or sour cream, chopped cilantro

Instructions:
1. Preheat your oven to 350°F (175°C).

2. In a large skillet, heat a bit of oil over medium heat. Add the diced onion and bell pepper. Cook for 3-4 minutes until softened.

3. Add the corn kernels, diced tomatoes, chili powder, ground cumin, smoked paprika, salt, and pepper to the skillet. Cook for another 2-3 minutes, stirring occasionally.

4. Add the black beans and cooked brown rice to the skillet. Stir to combine and cook for another 2-3 minutes until heated through. Taste and adjust seasoning if needed.

5. Place a portion of the bean and vegetable mixture onto each whole wheat tortilla, leaving a border around the edges. Sprinkle shredded cheese over the filling.

6. Fold the sides of each tortilla over the filling, then roll up tightly from the bottom to enclose the filling.

7. Place the rolled burritos seam-side down on a baking sheet lined with parchment paper or aluminum foil.

8. Bake the burritos in the preheated oven for 10-15 minutes, or until the tortillas are lightly crisp and the cheese is melted.

9. Remove the baked burritos from the oven and let them cool slightly before serving.

10. Serve the bean and vegetable burritos on whole wheat tortillas with your favorite toppings such as diced avocado, salsa, Greek yogurt or sour cream, and chopped cilantro.

23. Tilapia with mango salsa and steamed broccoli

Ingredients:
For the Tilapia:
- 4 tilapia fillets
- 1 tablespoon olive oil
- Salt and pepper to taste
- 1 teaspoon paprika
- 1 teaspoon garlic powder
- 1 teaspoon dried thyme (optional)

For the Steamed Broccoli:
- 2 heads of broccoli, cut into florets
- Salt to taste
- Lemon wedges for serving (optional)

For the Mango Salsa:
- 1 ripe mango, peeled, pitted, and diced
- 1/2 red bell pepper, diced
- 1/4 red onion, finely chopped
- 1 jalapeño pepper, seeded and minced (optional)
- Juice of 1 lime
- 2 tablespoons chopped fresh cilantro
- Salt and pepper to taste

Instructions:
1. Preheat your oven to 400°F (200°C).

2. Season the tilapia fillets with salt, pepper, paprika, garlic powder, and dried thyme (if using).

3. Heat olive oil in an oven-safe skillet over medium-high heat. Once hot, add the seasoned tilapia fillets to the skillet.

4. Sear the tilapia for 2-3 minutes on each side until lightly browned.

5. Transfer the skillet to the preheated oven and bake the tilapia for 8-10 minutes, or until it flakes easily with a fork.

6. While the tilapia is baking, prepare the mango salsa. In a bowl, combine diced mango, diced red bell pepper, finely chopped red onion, minced jalapeño pepper (if using), lime juice, chopped cilantro, salt, and pepper. Mix well and set aside.

7. Steam the broccoli florets until tender, about 5-7 minutes. Season with salt to taste.

8. Once the tilapia is cooked through, remove it from the oven.

9. Serve the tilapia fillets topped with mango salsa alongside steamed broccoli.

10. Optionally, serve with lemon wedges for squeezing over the fish and broccoli for added flavor.

24. Tofu veggie stir-fry over brown rice

Ingredients:

For the Tofu:
- 1 block (14 oz) firm tofu, pressed and cubed
- 2 tablespoons soy sauce
- 1 tablespoon cornstarch
- 1 tablespoon sesame oil
- 1 tablespoon olive oil

Optional toppings: sesame seeds, chopped green onions

For the Stir-Fry Sauce:
- 1/4 cup soy sauce
- 2 tablespoons hoisin sauce
- 1 tablespoon rice vinegar
- 1 tablespoon maple syrup or honey
- 2 cloves garlic, minced
- 1 teaspoon grated ginger
- 1 teaspoon sesame oil

For the Stir-Fry:
- 2 cups mixed vegetables (such as bell peppers, broccoli, carrots, snap peas)
- 1 onion, sliced
- 2 cloves garlic, minced
- 1 tablespoon olive oil
- Cooked brown rice for serving

Instructions:

1. Start by pressing the tofu to remove excess water. Place the tofu block between two paper towels or clean kitchen towels, then place a heavy object on top (like a cast-iron skillet). Let it press for about 20-30 minutes.

2. In a small bowl, whisk together the soy sauce, cornstarch, and sesame oil. Toss the cubed tofu in this mixture until evenly coated.

3. In another bowl, mix together all the ingredients for the stir-fry sauce: soy sauce, hoisin sauce, rice vinegar, maple syrup or honey, minced garlic, grated ginger, and sesame oil. Set aside.

4. Heat olive oil in a large skillet or wok over medium-high heat. Add the tofu cubes and cook until golden and crispy on all sides, about 5-7 minutes. Remove the tofu from the skillet and set aside.

5. In the same skillet, add another tablespoon of olive oil if needed. Add the sliced onion and minced garlic, and cook for 2-3 minutes until softened and fragrant.

6. Add the mixed vegetables to the skillet and stir-fry for 4-5 minutes until they are tender but still crisp.

7. Return the cooked tofu to the skillet with the vegetables. Pour the stir-fry sauce over the tofu and vegetables. Stir well to coat everything evenly. Cook for another 2-3 minutes until the sauce thickens slightly.

8. Serve the tofu veggie stir-fry over cooked brown rice. Garnish with sesame seeds and chopped green onions if desired.

25. Whole wheat pasta with lentil marinara sauce

Ingredients:
For the Lentil Marinara Sauce:
- 1 cup dry brown or green lentils,
rinsed and drained
- 2 tablespoons olive oil
- 1 onion, diced
- 2 cloves garlic, minced
- 1 carrot, diced
- 1 celery stalk, diced
- 1 bell pepper, diced
- 1 can (14 oz) diced tomatoes
- 1 can (6 oz) tomato paste
- 2 cups vegetable broth
- 1 teaspoon dried oregano
- 1 teaspoon dried basil
- 1/2 teaspoon dried thyme
- Salt and pepper to taste

For the Whole Wheat Pasta:
- 12 oz whole wheat pasta
(spaghetti, penne, or your
choice)
- Salt for boiling water

Optional toppings: grated
Parmesan cheese, chopped
fresh basil

Instructions:

1. In a large pot, heat olive oil over medium heat. Add diced onion, minced garlic, diced carrot, diced celery, and diced bell pepper. Cook for 5-7 minutes until the vegetables are softened.

2. Add the rinsed lentils to the pot, along with diced tomatoes, tomato paste, vegetable broth, dried oregano, dried basil, dried thyme, salt, and pepper. Stir to combine.

3. Bring the mixture to a boil, then reduce the heat to low. Cover and let the sauce simmer for about 20-25 minutes, stirring occasionally, until the lentils are tender and the sauce has thickened. If the sauce becomes too thick, you can add a bit more vegetable broth or water to reach your desired consistency.

4. While the sauce is simmering, cook the whole wheat pasta according to the package instructions in a large pot of salted boiling water until al dente. Drain the cooked pasta and set aside.

5. Once the lentil marinara sauce is ready, taste and adjust seasoning with more salt and pepper if needed.

6. Serve the cooked whole wheat pasta topped with the lentil marinara sauce. Garnish with grated Parmesan cheese and chopped fresh basil if desired.

26. Fresh fruit with nuts

Ingredients:

- Assorted fresh fruits (such as berries, grapes, apple slices, pear slices, kiwi, pineapple, melon, etc.)
- Assorted nuts (such as almonds, walnuts, cashews, pecans, pistachios, etc.)

Instructions:

1. Wash and prepare your choice of fresh fruits. Cut larger fruits into bite-sized pieces if needed.

2. Arrange the fresh fruit on a serving platter or in individual bowls.

3. Choose a variety of nuts to accompany the fruit. You can leave them whole or chop them if desired.

4. Sprinkle the nuts over the fresh fruit or serve them in a separate bowl alongside the fruit.

5. Serve immediately and enjoy the combination of sweet, juicy fruit with crunchy, flavorful nuts.

This simple snack or dessert is not only delicious but also provides a good balance of carbohydrates, fiber, healthy fats, and protein, making it a nutritious option for any time of day.

27. Veggie sticks with hummus or guacamole

Ingredients:

For the Guacamole:
- 2 ripe avocados
- 1 small tomato, diced
- 1/4 cup finely chopped onion
- 1/4 cup chopped fresh cilantro
- 1 jalapeño pepper, seeded and minced (optional)
- Juice of 1 lime
- Salt and pepper to taste

For the Veggie Sticks:
- Assorted fresh vegetables (such as carrots, celery, bell peppers, cucumber, cherry tomatoes, broccoli, cauliflower, etc.)

For the Hummus:
- 1 can (15 oz) chickpeas (garbanzo beans), drained and rinsed
- 2 tablespoons tahini (sesame seed paste)
- 2 tablespoons lemon juice
- 2 cloves garlic, minced
- 2 tablespoons olive oil
- Salt to taste
- Water (optional, for adjusting consistency)

Instructions:

1. Wash and prepare your choice of fresh vegetables. Cut them into sticks or slices for easy dipping.

2. To make the hummus, combine the drained and rinsed chickpeas, tahini, lemon juice, minced garlic, olive oil, and salt in a food processor. Blend until smooth, scraping down the sides as needed. If the hummus is too thick, you can add a little water, one tablespoon at a time, until you reach your desired consistency.

3. Transfer the hummus to a serving bowl and garnish with a drizzle of olive oil, a sprinkle of paprika, and some chopped fresh parsley if desired.

4. To make the guacamole, cut the avocados in half and remove the pits. Scoop the flesh into a bowl and mash it with a fork until smooth or chunky, depending on your preference.

5. Add the diced tomato, finely chopped onion, chopped cilantro, minced jalapeño pepper (if using), lime juice, salt, and pepper to the mashed avocado. Stir until well combined.

6. Taste the guacamole and adjust seasoning if needed.

7. Transfer the guacamole to a serving bowl and garnish with additional chopped cilantro and a sprinkle of paprika if desired.

8. Arrange the veggie sticks and bowls of hummus and guacamole on a serving platter. Serve the veggie sticks with hummus or guacamole for dipping.

28. Edamame

Ingredients:
- Edamame (frozen or fresh)
- Salt (optional, for seasoning)

Instructions:
1. If using frozen edamame, thaw it according to the package instructions. If using fresh edamame in the pod, rinse them under cold water.

2. Bring a pot of water to a boil. Add a pinch of salt if desired.

3. Add the edamame to the boiling water and cook for 3-5 minutes, or until they are tender.

4. Drain the cooked edamame and rinse them under cold water to stop the cooking process and cool them down.

5. Serve the edamame in a bowl, sprinkled with a little more salt if desired.

6. To eat, simply squeeze the beans out of the pods with your fingers or teeth. Discard the pods.

7. Enjoy the delicious and nutritious edamame as a snack, appetizer, or side dish.

Edamame is not only tasty but also packed with protein, fiber, vitamins, and minerals, making it a healthy addition to your diet.

29. Air-popped popcorn

Ingredients:
- 1/4 cup popcorn kernels
- Optional toppings: melted butter, olive oil, salt, nutritional yeast, herbs, spices, grated cheese, etc.

Instructions:

1. Place a large pot or popcorn popper on the stovetop over medium heat.

2. Add the popcorn kernels to the pot or popper.

3. Cover the pot with a lid or turn on the popcorn popper.

4. Let the kernels heat up, and they will start popping. Shake the pot occasionally to ensure even popping.

5. Once the popping slows down to about 2 seconds between pops, remove the pot from the heat or turn off the popcorn popper.

6. Carefully remove the lid, keeping it away from your face to avoid steam burns.

7. Transfer the air-popped popcorn to a large bowl.

8. If desired, drizzle melted butter or olive oil over the popcorn and toss to coat evenly.

9. Season the popcorn with salt, nutritional yeast, herbs, spices, grated cheese, or any other toppings you prefer. Toss again to distribute the toppings evenly.

10. Serve the air-popped popcorn immediately and enjoy!

Air-popped popcorn is a low-calorie snack that's high in fiber and whole grains. It's customizable with various toppings to suit your taste preferences. Plus, it's fun to make and delicious to eat!

30. Whole grain crackers with nut butter

Ingredients:
- Whole grain crackers (such as whole wheat, rye, or multigrain)
- Nut butter (such as peanut butter, almond butter, cashew butter, or sunflower seed butter)

Optional toppings:
- Sliced banana
- Apple slices
- Honey or maple syrup
- Chia seeds
- Flaxseeds
- Cinnamon

Instructions:

1. Spread a layer of nut butter onto each whole grain cracker.

2. If desired, top the nut butter with sliced banana, apple slices, or any other toppings of your choice.

3. Arrange the whole grain crackers with nut butter on a serving plate.

4. Serve immediately and enjoy your delicious and nutritious snack!

Whole grain crackers provide fiber and complex carbohydrates, while nut butter adds healthy fats, protein, and flavor. This snack is not only satisfying but also provides long-lasting energy to keep you fueled throughout the day. Feel free to customize it with your favorite toppings for extra flavor and nutrition!

31. Spinach salad with strawberries, pecans, and balsamic vinaigrette

Ingredients:
For the Salad:
- 6 cups fresh baby spinach leaves, washed and dried
- 1 cup fresh strawberries, hulled and sliced
- 1/2 cup pecans, toasted and chopped
- Optional additions: crumbled feta cheese, sliced red onion, avocado slices

For the Balsamic Vinaigrette:
- 1/4 cup balsamic vinegar
- 1/4 cup extra virgin olive oil
- 1 tablespoon honey or maple syrup
- 1 teaspoon Dijon mustard
- Salt and pepper to taste

Instructions:
1. In a large salad bowl, combine the fresh baby spinach leaves, sliced strawberries, and toasted chopped pecans. If using any optional additions like crumbled feta cheese, sliced red onion, or avocado slices, add them to the bowl as well.

2. In a small bowl or jar, whisk together the balsamic vinegar, extra virgin olive oil, honey or maple syrup, Dijon mustard, salt, and pepper until well combined. Alternatively, you can place all the vinaigrette ingredients in a jar with a tight-fitting lid and shake vigorously until emulsified.

3. Drizzle the balsamic vinaigrette over the salad, starting with a small amount and adding more to taste. Toss the salad gently to coat the ingredients evenly with the vinaigrette.

4. Serve the spinach salad with strawberries, pecans, and balsamic vinaigrette immediately as a refreshing appetizer or side dish.

5. Enjoy your delicious and nutritious salad!

This salad is perfect for spring and summer, with the sweetness of the strawberries complementing the earthy flavor of the spinach and the crunch of the toasted pecans. The balsamic vinaigrette adds a tangy and slightly sweet dressing that ties all the flavors together beautifully.

32. Quinoa tabbouleh salad

Ingredients:

For the Salad:
- 1 cup quinoa, rinsed
- 2 cups water or vegetable broth
- 1 cucumber, diced
- 2 tomatoes, diced
- 1/2 red onion, finely chopped
- 1/2 cup fresh parsley, chopped
- 1/4 cup fresh mint leaves, chopped
- 1/4 cup sliced black olives (optional)
- Salt and pepper to taste

For the Dressing:
- 1/4 cup extra virgin olive oil
- 2 tablespoons fresh lemon juice
- 1 clove garlic, minced
- 1 teaspoon ground cumin
- Salt and pepper to taste

Instructions:

1. In a medium saucepan, combine the quinoa and water or vegetable broth. Bring to a boil, then reduce the heat to low, cover, and simmer for 15-20 minutes, or until the quinoa is cooked and the liquid is absorbed. Remove from heat and let it cool.

2. While the quinoa is cooking, prepare the vegetables. Dice the cucumber, tomatoes, and red onion. Chop the fresh parsley and mint leaves.

3. In a large salad bowl, combine the cooked quinoa, diced cucumber, diced tomatoes, finely chopped red onion, chopped parsley, chopped mint leaves, and sliced black olives (if using). Season with salt and pepper to taste.

4. In a small bowl, whisk together the extra virgin olive oil, fresh lemon juice, minced garlic, ground cumin, salt, and pepper to make the dressing.

5. Pour the dressing over the quinoa tabbouleh salad and toss gently to coat all the ingredients evenly with the dressing.

6. Taste and adjust seasoning if needed.

7. Chill the salad in the refrigerator for at least 30 minutes to allow the flavors to meld together.

8. Serve the quinoa tabbouleh salad chilled as a refreshing and nutritious side dish or light meal.

33. Black bean and corn salad

Ingredients:
- 2 cans (15 oz each) black beans, drained and rinsed
- 2 cups frozen corn kernels, thawed
- 1 red bell pepper, diced
- 1/2 red onion, finely chopped
- 1/4 cup fresh cilantro, chopped
- Juice of 2 limes
- 2 tablespoons olive oil
- 1 teaspoon ground cumin
- 1/2 teaspoon chili powder
- Salt and pepper to taste
- Optional toppings: diced avocado, crumbled feta or cotija cheese, sliced jalapeños, chopped green onions

Instructions:

1. In a large mixing bowl, combine the black beans, thawed corn kernels, diced red bell pepper, finely chopped red onion, and chopped fresh cilantro.

2. In a small bowl, whisk together the lime juice, olive oil, ground cumin, chili powder, salt, and pepper to make the dressing.

3. Pour the dressing over the black bean and corn mixture in the large bowl.

4. Toss everything together until well combined and evenly coated with the dressing.

5. Taste and adjust seasoning if needed.

6. If desired, add any optional toppings such as diced avocado, crumbled feta or cotija cheese, sliced jalapeños, or chopped green onions.

7. Chill the black bean and corn salad in the refrigerator for at least 30 minutes to allow the flavors to meld together.

8. Serve the salad chilled as a side dish or appetizer, or enjoy it as a light and refreshing meal on its own.

This black bean and corn salad is packed with flavor, fiber, and protein, making it both delicious and nutritious. Enjoy its vibrant colors and fresh taste!

34. Kale caesar salad with baked chicken

Ingredients:
For the Baked Chicken:
- 2 boneless, skinless chicken breasts
- 1 tablespoon olive oil
- 1 teaspoon garlic powder
- 1 teaspoon smoked paprika
- Salt and pepper to taste

For the Kale Caesar Salad:
- 1 large bunch of kale, stems removed and leaves chopped
- 1/2 cup Caesar dressing (store-bought or homemade)
- 1/4 cup grated Parmesan cheese
- 1/2 cup croutons (store-bought or homemade)
- Lemon wedges for serving (optional)

Instructions:
1. Preheat your oven to 375°F (190°C).

2. Place the boneless, skinless chicken breasts on a baking sheet lined with parchment paper or aluminum foil.

3. Drizzle the olive oil over the chicken breasts and sprinkle with garlic powder, smoked paprika, salt, and pepper, rubbing the seasoning evenly over both sides of the chicken.

4. Bake the chicken in the preheated oven for 20-25 minutes, or until cooked through and no longer pink in the center. The internal temperature should reach 165°F (75°C). Once cooked, remove the chicken from the oven and let it rest for a few minutes before slicing.

5. While the chicken is baking, prepare the kale Caesar salad. In a large mixing bowl, combine the chopped kale leaves and Caesar dressing. Use your hands to massage the dressing into the kale leaves for a minute or two, which helps to tenderize the kale.

6. Add the grated Parmesan cheese and croutons to the bowl with the dressed kale, and toss to combine.

7. Divide the kale Caesar salad among serving plates.

8. Slice the baked chicken breasts and arrange them on top of the salad. Serve the kale Caesar salad with baked chicken immediately, with lemon wedges on the side for squeezing over the chicken if desired

35. Greek salad with chickpeas

Ingredients:
For the Salad:
- 1 can (15 oz) chickpeas (garbanzo beans), drained and rinsed
- 1 English cucumber, diced
- 2 large tomatoes, diced
- 1 red bell pepper, diced
- 1/2 red onion, thinly sliced
- 1/2 cup Kalamata olives, pitted
- 1/2 cup crumbled feta cheese
- 1/4 cup chopped fresh parsley
- Optional: 1/4 cup chopped fresh mint leaves

For the Dressing:
- 1/4 cup extra virgin olive oil
- 2 tablespoons red wine vinegar
- 1 clove garlic, minced
- 1 teaspoon dried oregano
- Salt and pepper to taste

Instructions:
1. In a large salad bowl, combine the chickpeas, diced cucumber, diced tomatoes, diced red bell pepper, thinly sliced red onion, pitted Kalamata olives, crumbled feta cheese, chopped fresh parsley, and chopped fresh mint leaves (if using).

2. In a small bowl or jar, whisk together the extra virgin olive oil, red wine vinegar, minced garlic, dried oregano, salt, and pepper to make the dressing.

3. Pour the dressing over the salad ingredients in the large bowl.

4. Toss everything together until well combined and evenly coated with the dressing.

5. Taste and adjust seasoning if needed.

6. Chill the Greek salad with chickpeas in the refrigerator for at least 30 minutes to allow the flavors to meld together. Serve the salad chilled as a refreshing and nutritious side dish or light meal.

This Greek salad with chickpeas is packed with protein, fiber, and Mediterranean flavors. It's perfect for picnics, potlucks, or as a healthy lunch option. Enjoy its vibrant colors and delicious taste!

36. Butternut squash soup

Ingredients:
- 1 medium butternut squash (about 2-3 pounds), peeled, seeded, and cubed
- 1 onion, diced
- 2 carrots, diced
- 2 stalks celery, diced
- 2 cloves garlic, minced
- 4 cups vegetable broth
- 1 teaspoon dried thyme
- 1/2 teaspoon ground cinnamon
- 1/4 teaspoon ground nutmeg
- Salt and pepper to taste
- 2 tablespoons olive oil or butter
- Optional garnishes: chopped fresh parsley, toasted pumpkin seeds, a drizzle of cream or coconut milk

Instructions:
1. Heat the olive oil or butter in a large pot over medium heat. Add the diced onion, carrots, and celery. Cook for 5-7 minutes until the vegetables are softened.

2. Add the minced garlic to the pot and cook for another minute until fragrant.

3. Add the cubed butternut squash to the pot, along with the vegetable broth, dried thyme, ground cinnamon, and ground nutmeg. Bring the mixture to a boil.

4. Once boiling, reduce the heat to low, cover the pot, and let the soup simmer for about 20-25 minutes, or until the butternut squash is tender.

5. Once the butternut squash is tender, remove the pot from the heat. Use an immersion blender to puree the soup until smooth and creamy. Alternatively, you can carefully transfer the soup in batches to a blender and blend until smooth, then return it to the pot.

6. Taste the soup and season with salt and pepper according to your preference.

7. If the soup is too thick, you can add more vegetable broth or water to reach your desired consistency.

8. Return the pot to the stove and heat the soup over low heat until warmed through.

9. Serve the butternut squash soup hot, garnished with chopped fresh parsley, toasted pumpkin seeds, and a drizzle of cream or coconut milk if desired.

37. Split pea soup

Ingredients:
- 1 lb (about 2 cups) dried green split peas, rinsed and picked over
- 1 ham bone, ham hock, or 1 cup diced cooked ham (optional)
- 2 carrots, diced
- 2 stalks celery, diced
- 1 onion, diced
- 2 cloves garlic, minced
- 6 cups vegetable or chicken broth
- 2 bay leaves
- 1 teaspoon dried thyme
- Salt and pepper to taste
- 2 tablespoons olive oil or butter
- Optional toppings: chopped fresh parsley, croutons, sour cream or yogurt

Instructions:
1. In a large pot or Dutch oven, heat the olive oil or butter over medium heat. Add the diced onion, carrots, and celery. Cook for 5-7 minutes until the vegetables are softened.

2. Add the minced garlic to the pot and cook for another minute until fragrant.

3. Add the rinsed split peas, ham bone or ham hock (if using), bay leaves, dried thyme, and vegetable or chicken broth to the pot. Stir to combine.

4. Bring the mixture to a boil, then reduce the heat to low. Cover the pot and let the soup simmer for about 1 to 1 1/2 hours, stirring occasionally, or until the split peas are tender and the soup has thickened.

5. If using a ham bone or ham hock, remove it from the soup and let it cool slightly. Once cool enough to handle, remove any meat from the bone, chop it, and return it to the soup. If using diced cooked ham, add it to the soup.

6. Taste the soup and season with salt and pepper according to your preference.

7. If the soup is too thick, you can add more broth or water to reach your desired consistency.

8. Remove the bay leaves from the soup before serving.

9. Serve the split pea soup hot, garnished with chopped fresh parsley, croutons, sour cream or yogurt if desired.

38. Vegetable barley soup

Ingredients:
- 1 cup pearl barley, rinsed
- 1 tablespoon olive oil
- 1 onion, diced
- 2 carrots, diced
- 2 celery stalks, diced
- 2 cloves garlic, minced
- 1 bell pepper, diced
- 1 zucchini, diced
- 1 can (14 oz) diced tomatoes
- 6 cups vegetable broth
- 2 bay leaves
- 1 teaspoon dried thyme
- Salt and pepper to taste
- Chopped fresh parsley for garnish (optional)

Instructions:
1. In a large pot or Dutch oven, heat the olive oil over medium heat. Add the diced onion, carrots, and celery. Cook for about 5 minutes until the vegetables are softened.

2. Add the minced garlic to the pot and cook for another minute until fragrant.

3. Add the diced bell pepper and zucchini to the pot, and cook for another 3-4 minutes until they start to soften.

4. Stir in the rinsed pearl barley, diced tomatoes (with their juices), vegetable broth, bay leaves, and dried thyme. Bring the soup to a boil.

5. Once boiling, reduce the heat to low. Cover the pot and let the soup simmer for about 30-40 minutes, stirring occasionally, or until the barley is tender.

6. Taste the soup and season with salt and pepper according to your preference.

7. If the soup is too thick, you can add more vegetable broth or water to reach your desired consistency.

8. Remove the bay leaves from the soup before serving.

9. Serve the vegetable barley soup hot, garnished with chopped fresh parsley if desired.

39. White bean and kale soup

Ingredients:
- 1 tablespoon olive oil
- 1 onion, diced
- 2 carrots, diced
- 2 celery stalks, diced
- 3 cloves garlic, minced
- 4 cups vegetable broth
- 2 cans (15 oz each) white beans (such as cannellini or navy beans), drained and rinsed
- 1 can (14 oz) diced tomatoes
- 1 teaspoon dried thyme
- 1 teaspoon dried rosemary
- 1 bay leaf
- Salt and pepper to taste
- 4 cups chopped kale leaves (stems removed)
- 1 tablespoon lemon juice
- Grated Parmesan cheese for serving (optional)

Instructions:
1. In a large pot or Dutch oven, heat the olive oil over medium heat. Add the diced onion, carrots, and celery. Cook for about 5 minutes until the vegetables are softened.

2. Add the minced garlic to the pot and cook for another minute until fragrant.

3. Stir in the vegetable broth, white beans, diced tomatoes (with their juices), dried thyme, dried rosemary, and bay leaf. Bring the soup to a boil.

4. Once boiling, reduce the heat to low. Cover the pot and let the soup simmer for about 20-25 minutes, stirring occasionally.

5. Taste the soup and season with salt and pepper according to your preference.

6. Add the chopped kale leaves to the pot and stir until wilted, about 5 minutes.

7. Stir in the lemon juice.

8. Remove the bay leaf from the soup before serving.

9. Serve the white bean and kale soup hot, garnished with grated Parmesan cheese if desired.

40. Tomato basil soup

Ingredients:
- 2 tablespoons olive oil
- 1 onion, diced
- 2 cloves garlic, minced
- 2 cans (28 oz each) whole peeled tomatoes
- 1 cup vegetable broth
- 1/2 cup fresh basil leaves, chopped
- 1 teaspoon dried oregano
- 1/2 teaspoon dried thyme
- Salt and pepper to taste
- 1/4 cup heavy cream (optional, for added richness)
- Grated Parmesan cheese for serving (optional)

Instructions:
1. In a large pot or Dutch oven, heat the olive oil over medium heat. Add the diced onion and cook until softened, about 5 minutes.

2. Add the minced garlic to the pot and cook for another minute until fragrant.

3. Add the canned whole peeled tomatoes (with their juices) to the pot, breaking them up with a spoon or spatula. Stir in the vegetable broth, chopped fresh basil, dried oregano, and dried thyme.

4. Bring the soup to a simmer, then reduce the heat to low. Cover the pot and let the soup simmer for about 20-25 minutes, stirring occasionally.

5. Taste the soup and season with salt and pepper according to your preference.

6. If using, stir in the heavy cream to add richness to the soup.

7. Use an immersion blender to puree the soup until smooth and creamy. Alternatively, carefully transfer the soup in batches to a blender and blend until smooth, then return it to the pot.

8. Once the soup is smooth and creamy, return it to the stove and heat over low heat until warmed through.

9. Serve the tomato basil soup hot, garnished with grated Parmesan cheese if desired.

41. Roasted brussels sprouts with balsamic glaze

Ingredients:
- 1 lb Brussels sprouts, trimmed and halved
- 2 tablespoons olive oil
- Salt and pepper to taste
- 2 tablespoons balsamic vinegar
- 1 tablespoon honey or maple syrup (optional, for added sweetness)
- Optional toppings: grated Parmesan cheese, chopped fresh parsley, toasted nuts (such as pecans or walnuts)

Instructions:
1. Preheat your oven to 400°F (200°C) and line a baking sheet with parchment paper or aluminum foil for easy cleanup.

2. In a large bowl, toss the halved Brussels sprouts with olive oil, salt, and pepper until evenly coated.

3. Spread the Brussels sprouts out in a single layer on the prepared baking sheet.

4. Roast the Brussels sprouts in the preheated oven for 20-25 minutes, or until they are tender and caramelized, stirring halfway through to ensure even cooking.

5. While the Brussels sprouts are roasting, prepare the balsamic glaze. In a small saucepan, combine the balsamic vinegar and honey or maple syrup (if using). Bring the mixture to a simmer over medium heat, then reduce the heat to low and let it cook for 5-7 minutes, stirring occasionally, until it thickens and reduces by about half. Remove from heat.

6. Once the Brussels sprouts are roasted to your liking, remove them from the oven and transfer them to a serving dish.

7. Drizzle the balsamic glaze over the roasted Brussels sprouts, tossing gently to coat.

8. If desired, garnish the Brussels sprouts with grated Parmesan cheese, chopped fresh parsley, or toasted nuts before serving.

9. Serve the roasted Brussels sprouts with balsamic glaze immediately as a delicious side dish.

Enjoy your flavorful and caramelized roasted Brussels sprouts with balsamic glaze!

42. Grilled vegetable kabobs

Ingredients:
- Assorted vegetables, such as bell peppers, zucchini, yellow squash, cherry tomatoes, red onions, mushrooms, etc.
- Olive oil
- Balsamic vinegar (optional)
- Garlic powder
- Dried herbs, such as thyme, oregano, or basil
- Salt and pepper to taste
- Wooden or metal skewers

Instructions:
1. If you're using wooden skewers, soak them in water for at least 30 minutes to prevent them from burning on the grill.

2. Prepare your assortment of vegetables by washing and cutting them into bite-sized pieces. Try to cut them into similar-sized pieces so they cook evenly on the grill.

3. In a large bowl, toss the vegetables with olive oil, balsamic vinegar (if using), garlic powder, dried herbs, salt, and pepper. You can adjust the seasonings to your taste preferences.

4. Thread the seasoned vegetables onto the skewers, alternating between different types of vegetables to create colorful kabobs.

5. Preheat your grill to medium-high heat.

6. Place the vegetable kabobs on the grill, and cook for 10-15 minutes, turning occasionally, until the vegetables are tender and slightly charred.

7. Once the kabobs are cooked to your liking, remove them from the grill and transfer them to a serving platter.

8. Serve the grilled vegetable kabobs hot as a delicious side dish or main course.

Enjoy your flavorful and colorful grilled vegetable kabobs!

43. Spaghetti squash with marinara sauce

Ingredients:
- 1 medium spaghetti squash
- Olive oil
- Salt and pepper to taste
- Marinara sauce (homemade or store-bought)
- Grated Parmesan cheese (optional)
- Chopped fresh basil or parsley for garnish (optional)

Instructions:
1. Preheat your oven to 400°F (200°C).

2. Wash the spaghetti squash and carefully cut it in half lengthwise using a sharp knife. Be cautious, as spaghetti squash can be quite firm and challenging to cut. You can also poke holes in the squash and microwave it for a few minutes to soften it slightly before cutting.

3. Scoop out the seeds and stringy pulp from the center of the spaghetti squash halves using a spoon.

4. Drizzle the cut sides of the spaghetti squash halves with olive oil and season with salt and pepper.

5. Place the spaghetti squash halves, cut side down, on a baking sheet lined with parchment paper or aluminum foil.

6. Roast the spaghetti squash in the preheated oven for 35-45 minutes, or until the flesh is tender and easily pierced with a fork.

7. Once the spaghetti squash is cooked, remove it from the oven and let it cool slightly until it's safe to handle.

8. Use a fork to scrape the cooked flesh of the spaghetti squash into strands, resembling spaghetti noodles. Transfer the spaghetti squash "noodles" to a serving dish.

9. Heat the marinara sauce in a saucepan over medium heat until warmed through.

10. Pour the marinara sauce over the spaghetti squash "noodles" and toss gently to coat.

11. If desired, sprinkle grated Parmesan cheese and chopped fresh basil or parsley over the top for added flavor and garnish. Serve the spaghetti squash with marinara sauce hot as a delicious and nutritious meal.

44. Stuffed bell peppers with quinoa and veggies

Ingredients:
- 4 large bell peppers (any color), tops removed and seeds removed
- 1 cup cooked quinoa
- 1 tablespoon olive oil
- 1 onion, diced
- 2 cloves garlic, minced
- 2 carrots, diced
- 2 stalks celery, diced
- 1 zucchini, diced
- 1 cup diced tomatoes (fresh or canned)
- 1 teaspoon dried oregano
- 1 teaspoon dried basil
- Salt and pepper to taste
- 1/2 cup shredded cheese (such as mozzarella or cheddar)
- Optional toppings: chopped fresh parsley, grated Parmesan cheese

Instructions:
1. Preheat your oven to 375°F (190°C).

2. In a large skillet, heat the olive oil over medium heat. Add the diced onion and cook until softened, about 5 minutes.

3. Add the minced garlic to the skillet and cook for another minute until fragrant. Stir in the diced carrots, celery, and zucchini. Cook for 5-7 minutes until the vegetables are tender.

4. Add the diced tomatoes, dried oregano, dried basil, cooked quinoa, salt, and pepper to the skillet. Stir to combine and cook for another 2-3 minutes to allow the flavors to meld together.

5. Remove the skillet from the heat and let the filling mixture cool slightly. Spoon the filling mixture into the hollowed-out bell peppers, packing it tightly.

6. Place the stuffed bell peppers upright in a baking dish. If the bell peppers don't stand up straight, you can slice a thin piece off the bottom to create a flat surface.

7. Sprinkle shredded cheese over the top of each stuffed bell pepper. Cover the baking dish with aluminum foil and bake in the preheated oven for 25-30 minutes.

8. Remove the foil and bake for an additional 5-10 minutes, or until the cheese is melted and bubbly, and the bell peppers are tender.

9. Once cooked, remove the stuffed bell peppers from the oven and let them cool for a few minutes before serving.

10. Serve the stuffed bell peppers with quinoa and veggies hot, garnished with chopped fresh parsley or grated Parmesan cheese if desired.

45. Roasted beet and arugula salad

Ingredients:
For the Roasted Beets:
- 3-4 medium beets, washed and trimmed
- Olive oil
- Salt and pepper to taste

For the Salad:
- 4 cups fresh arugula leaves, washed and dried
- 1/4 cup crumbled goat cheese or feta cheese
- 1/4 cup chopped walnuts or pecans, toasted
- Balsamic glaze or vinaigrette dressing

Instructions:
1. Preheat your oven to 400°F (200°C).

2. Place the washed and trimmed beets on a large sheet of aluminum foil. Drizzle them with olive oil and season with salt and pepper.

3. Wrap the beets tightly in the aluminum foil, forming a packet.

4. Place the foil packet on a baking sheet and roast the beets in the preheated oven for 45-60 minutes, or until they are fork-tender.

5. Once the beets are cooked, remove them from the oven and let them cool slightly until they are safe to handle.

6. Peel the skins off the roasted beets using your fingers or a paper towel. The skins should slide off easily.

7. Cut the peeled roasted beets into wedges or slices. In a large salad bowl, combine the fresh arugula leaves with the roasted beet wedges or slices.

8. Sprinkle crumbled goat cheese or feta cheese and chopped toasted walnuts or pecans over the top of the salad.

9. Drizzle balsamic glaze or vinaigrette dressing over the salad, tossing gently to coat all the ingredients evenly.

10. Taste and adjust seasoning if needed. Serve the roasted beet and arugula salad immediately as a colorful and flavorful appetizer or side dish.

46. Cauliflower rice stir fry

Ingredients:
- 1 head of cauliflower
- 2 tablespoons sesame oil or olive oil
- 2 cloves garlic, minced
- 1 small onion, diced
- 1 carrot, diced
- 1 bell pepper, diced
- 1 cup chopped broccoli florets
- 1 cup chopped mushrooms
- 1 cup frozen peas, thawed
- 2-3 tablespoons soy sauce or tamari
- 1 tablespoon rice vinegar
- 1 teaspoon grated fresh ginger (optional)
- Salt and pepper to taste
- Green onions, chopped, for garnish (optional)
- Sesame seeds, for garnish (optional)

Instructions:

1. Wash the cauliflower and remove the leaves and tough stem. Cut the cauliflower into florets.

2. Place the cauliflower florets in a food processor and pulse until they resemble the texture of rice or couscous. Be careful not to over-process, or it will turn into a puree.

3. Heat 1 tablespoon of sesame oil or olive oil in a large skillet or wok over medium heat. Add the minced garlic and diced onion, and sauté until softened and fragrant, about 2-3 minutes.

4. Add the diced carrot, bell pepper, broccoli florets, and mushrooms to the skillet. Cook, stirring frequently, for about 5-7 minutes, or until the vegetables are tender-crisp.

5. Push the vegetables to one side of the skillet and add the remaining tablespoon of sesame oil or olive oil to the empty space. Add the riced cauliflower to the skillet and stir-fry for 3-4 minutes, or until it is heated through and tender.

6. Stir in the thawed peas, soy sauce or tamari, rice vinegar, and grated fresh ginger (if using). Cook for another 2-3 minutes, stirring constantly, until everything is well combined and heated through.

7. Taste the cauliflower rice stir-fry and adjust the seasoning with salt and pepper as needed.

8. Garnish the stir-fry with chopped green onions and sesame seeds if desired. Serve the cauliflower rice stir-fry hot as a delicious and healthy meal or side dish.

47. Zucchini noodles with pesto

For the Zucchini Noodles:
- 4 medium zucchini
- Salt

For the Pesto:
- 2 cups fresh basil leaves, packed
- 1/3 cup pine nuts or walnuts
- 2 cloves garlic, minced
- 1/2 cup grated Parmesan cheese
- 1/2 cup extra virgin olive oil
- Salt and pepper to taste

Instructions:

1. Wash the zucchini and trim off the ends. Using a spiralizer, julienne peeler, or mandoline slicer, cut the zucchini into long, thin noodle-like strips. Alternatively, you can use a knife to slice the zucchini into thin strips resembling noodles.

2. Place the zucchini noodles in a colander set over a bowl or in the sink. Sprinkle the noodles with salt and toss to coat. Let the noodles sit for about 10-15 minutes to release excess moisture.

3. While the zucchini noodles are draining, prepare the pesto. In a food processor, combine the fresh basil leaves, pine nuts or walnuts, minced garlic, and grated Parmesan cheese. Pulse until the ingredients are finely chopped.

4. With the food processor running, slowly drizzle in the olive oil until the pesto reaches your desired consistency. Season with salt and pepper to taste, and pulse to combine.

5. After the zucchini noodles have drained, use paper towels or a clean kitchen towel to gently squeeze out any excess moisture.

6. Heat a large skillet over medium heat. Add the zucchini noodles to the skillet and cook, tossing frequently, for 2-3 minutes, or until the noodles are heated through and slightly softened.

7. Remove the skillet from the heat and add the pesto to the zucchini noodles. Toss gently to coat the noodles evenly with the pesto.

8. Taste the zucchini noodles with pesto and adjust the seasoning with salt and pepper if needed. Serve the zucchini noodles with pesto immediately as a light and flavorful meal.

48. Butternut squash and kale hash

Ingredients:
- 1 teaspoon dried thyme
- 1/2 teaspoon smoked paprika (optional)
- Salt and pepper to taste
- 2-4 eggs (optional)
- Chopped fresh parsley for garnish (optional)

- 1 medium butternut squash, peeled and diced into small cubes
- 2 tablespoons olive oil
- 1 onion, diced
- 2 cloves garlic, minced
- 1 red bell pepper, diced
- 1 bunch kale, stems removed and leaves chopped

Instructions:

1. Preheat your oven to 400°F (200°C).

2. Spread the diced butternut squash on a baking sheet. Drizzle with 1 tablespoon of olive oil and season with salt and pepper. Toss to coat evenly.

3. Roast the butternut squash in the preheated oven for 25-30 minutes, or until tender and lightly browned, stirring halfway through.

4. While the butternut squash is roasting, heat the remaining 1 tablespoon of olive oil in a large skillet over medium heat. Add the diced onion and cook until softened, about 5 minutes.

5. Add the minced garlic and diced red bell pepper to the skillet. Cook for another 2-3 minutes until the vegetables are tender and fragrant.

6. Stir in the chopped kale, dried thyme, and smoked paprika (if using). Cook for about 5 minutes, or until the kale is wilted and tender.

7. Once the butternut squash is done roasting, add it to the skillet with the vegetables. Toss everything together and cook for another 2-3 minutes to allow the flavors to meld.

8. Taste the hash and season with additional salt and pepper if needed.

9. If you want to add eggs, create small wells in the hash and crack the eggs into the wells. Cover the skillet and cook until the eggs are done to your liking, about 5-7 minutes for set whites and runny yolks, or longer if you prefer fully cooked yolks.

10. Garnish the butternut squash and kale hash with chopped fresh parsley if desired. Serve the hash hot, with or without eggs, as a delicious and nutritious meal.

49. Eggplant rollatini with ricotta and spinach

Ingredients:
- 2 large eggplants
- Salt
- Olive oil
- 2 cups ricotta cheese
- 1 cup fresh spinach, chopped
- 1/2 cup grated Parmesan cheese
- 2 cloves garlic, minced
- 1 egg, beaten
- 1 teaspoon dried basil
- 1 teaspoon dried oregano
- 2 cups marinara sauce (homemade or store-bought)
- 1 cup shredded mozzarella cheese
- Fresh basil or parsley for garnish (optional)

Instructions:

1. Preheat your oven to 375°F (190°C).

2. Slice the eggplants lengthwise into 1/4-inch thick slices. Sprinkle both sides of the slices with salt and let them sit in a colander for about 20-30 minutes to draw out excess moisture and bitterness.

3. Rinse the eggplant slices under cold water and pat them dry with paper towels.

4. Brush both sides of the eggplant slices lightly with olive oil and place them on a baking sheet lined with parchment paper. Bake the eggplant slices in the preheated oven for about 15-20 minutes, or until they are tender and pliable. Remove from the oven and let them cool slightly.

5. While the eggplant slices are baking, prepare the ricotta filling. In a large bowl, combine the ricotta cheese, chopped spinach, grated Parmesan cheese, beaten egg, minced garlic, dried basil, and dried oregano. Mix well and season with salt and pepper to taste.

6. Spread a thin layer of marinara sauce on the bottom of a baking dish.

7. Take one eggplant slice and place a spoonful of the ricotta and spinach filling at one end. Roll the eggplant slice around the filling and place it seam-side down in the baking dish. Repeat with the remaining eggplant slices and filling.

8. Once all the eggplant rollatini are assembled in the baking dish, pour the remaining marinara sauce over the top of the rolls. Sprinkle the shredded mozzarella cheese evenly over the top.

9. Cover the baking dish with aluminum foil and bake in the preheated oven for 20 minutes. Remove the foil and bake for an additional 10-15 minutes, or until the cheese is melted and bubbly.

10. Remove the eggplant rollatini from the oven and let them cool for a few minutes before serving. Garnish with fresh basil or parsley if desired, and serve hot

50. Vegetarian chili

Ingredients:
- 2 tablespoons olive oil
- 1 large onion, diced
- 3 cloves garlic, minced
- 1 red bell pepper, diced
- 1 green bell pepper, diced
- 2 carrots, diced
- 2 celery stalks, diced
- 1 zucchini, diced
- 1 yellow squash, diced
- 1 jalapeño, seeded and minced
- 2 tablespoons chili powder
- 1 tablespoon ground cumin
- 1 teaspoon smoked paprika
- 1/2 teaspoon dried oregano
- 1/2 teaspoon ground coriander
- Salt and pepper to taste
- 1 can (28 oz) diced tomatoes
- 1 can (15 oz) tomato sauce
- 1 can (15 oz) black beans, drained and rinsed
- 1 can (15 oz) kidney beans, drained and rinsed
- 1 can (15 oz) pinto beans, drained and rinsed
- 1 cup vegetable broth
- 1 cup corn kernels (fresh or frozen)
- Juice of 1 lime
- Fresh cilantro, chopped, for garnish
- Sour cream or Greek yogurt, for serving (optional)
- Shredded cheddar cheese, for serving (optional)
- Sliced green onions, for garnish (optional)

Instructions:

1. In a large pot or Dutch oven, heat the olive oil over medium heat. Add the diced onion and cook until softened, about 5 minutes.

2. Add the minced garlic, red and green bell peppers, carrots, and celery. Cook for another 5-7 minutes until the vegetables begin to soften.

3. Stir in the diced zucchini, yellow squash, and minced jalapeño (if using). Cook for another 5 minutes, stirring occasionally.

4. Add the chili powder, ground cumin, smoked paprika, dried oregano, ground coriander, salt, and pepper. Stir to coat the vegetables with the spices and cook for about 1 minute until fragrant.

5. Add the diced tomatoes, tomato sauce, black beans, kidney beans, pinto beans, and vegetable broth to the pot. Stir well to combine.

6. Bring the chili to a simmer, then reduce the heat to low. Cover the pot and let the chili simmer for about 30-45 minutes, stirring occasionally to prevent sticking.

7. Stir in the corn kernels and cook for another 5-10 minutes until heated through. Remove the chili from the heat and stir in the lime juice. Taste and adjust seasoning with additional salt and pepper if needed.

8. Serve the vegetarian chili hot, garnished with chopped fresh cilantro, a dollop of sour cream or Greek yogurt, shredded cheddar cheese, and sliced green onions if desired.

51. Turkey meatballs in marinara sauce

Ingredients:

For the Turkey Meatballs:
- 1 lb ground turkey (preferably lean)
- 1/2 cup breadcrumbs
- 1/4 cup grated Parmesan cheese
- 1 egg, lightly beaten
- 2 cloves garlic, minced
- 1 tablespoon chopped fresh parsley
- 1 teaspoon dried oregano
- 1/2 teaspoon dried basil
- 1/2 teaspoon salt
- 1/4 teaspoon black pepper

For the Marinara Sauce:
- 2 tablespoons olive oil
- 1 onion, finely diced
- 2 cloves garlic, minced
- 1 can (28 oz) crushed tomatoes
- 1 can (14 oz) diced tomatoes
- 1 teaspoon dried basil
- 1 teaspoon dried oregano
- 1/2 teaspoon dried thyme
- Salt and pepper to taste
- Pinch of sugar (optional, to balance acidity)

Instructions:

1. Preheat your oven to 400°F (200°C). Line a baking sheet with parchment paper or aluminum foil for easy cleanup.

2. In a large bowl, combine the ground turkey, breadcrumbs, grated Parmesan cheese, beaten egg, minced garlic, chopped fresh parsley, dried oregano, dried basil, salt, and black pepper. Mix until well combined.

3. Shape the turkey mixture into meatballs, using about 1-2 tablespoons of mixture for each meatball. Place the meatballs on the prepared baking sheet, leaving a little space between each one.

4. Bake the turkey meatballs in the preheated oven for 20-25 minutes, or until they are cooked through and lightly browned.

5. While the meatballs are baking, prepare the marinara sauce. In a large skillet or saucepan, heat the olive oil over medium heat. Add the finely diced onion and cook until softened, about 5 minutes.

6. Add the minced garlic to the skillet and cook for another minute until fragrant. Stir in the crushed tomatoes, diced tomatoes (with their juices), dried basil, dried oregano, dried thyme, salt, pepper, and a pinch of sugar if using. Bring the sauce to a simmer.

7. Once the sauce is simmering, reduce the heat to low and let it simmer gently for about 15-20 minutes, stirring occasionally, to allow the flavors to meld together.

8. Once the meatballs are done baking and the marinara sauce is ready, add the meatballs to the skillet with the marinara sauce. Gently toss to coat the meatballs in the sauce.

9. Let the meatballs simmer in the sauce for another 5-10 minutes to absorb the flavors. Serve the turkey meatballs in marinara sauce hot, garnished with additional chopped parsley or grated Parmesan cheese if desired.

52. Baked tofu with teriyaki glaze

Ingredients:
- 1 block (14-16 oz) extra firm tofu
- 2 tbsp soy sauce or tamari
- 1 tbsp sesame oil
- 1 tbsp rice vinegar
- 1 tbsp maple syrup or honey
- 1 clove garlic, minced
- 1 tsp grated fresh ginger
- Sesame seeds and chopped green onions for garnish (optional)

For the Teriyaki Glaze:
- 1/4 cup soy sauce or tamari
- 2 tbsp mirin
- 2 tbsp rice vinegar
- 2 tbsp maple syrup or honey
- 1 clove garlic, minced
- 1 tsp grated fresh ginger
- 1 tsp cornstarch or arrowroot powder mixed with 1 tbsp water (optional)

Instructions:
1. Preheat oven to 400°F (200°C) and line a baking sheet.

2. Press tofu to remove excess moisture, then cut into cubes or slices.

3. Mix tofu with soy sauce, sesame oil, rice vinegar, maple syrup, garlic, and ginger. Marinate for 15-20 minutes.

4. Bake tofu for 25-30 minutes, flipping halfway through.

5. While tofu bakes, make the teriyaki glaze by simmering ingredients in a saucepan.

6. Optional: thicken glaze with cornstarch or arrowroot powder.

7. Once tofu is done, brush or drizzle with teriyaki glaze.

8. Garnish with sesame seeds and green onions if desired. Serve hot with rice and vegetables.

53. Lemon dill salmon packets

Ingredients:
- 4 salmon fillets (about 6 oz each)
- Salt and pepper to taste
- 2 lemons, thinly sliced
- 4 sprigs fresh dill
- 4 tablespoons butter or olive oil
- 4 cloves garlic, minced
- 4 teaspoons Dijon mustard
- Aluminum foil

Instructions:
1. Preheat your oven to 375°F (190°C).

2. Place each salmon fillet on a piece of aluminum foil large enough to wrap around it.

3. Season the salmon fillets with salt and pepper to taste.

4. Place 2-3 slices of lemon on top of each salmon fillet.

5. Add a sprig of fresh dill on top of the lemon slices.

6. In a small saucepan, melt the butter (or heat the olive oil) over medium heat. Add the minced garlic and cook for 1-2 minutes until fragrant.

7. Remove the saucepan from the heat and stir in the Dijon mustard until well combined.

8. Spoon the garlic mustard mixture evenly over the salmon fillets.

9. Fold the aluminum foil over the salmon fillets to create packets, making sure to seal the edges tightly.

10. Place the salmon packets on a baking sheet and bake in the preheated oven for 12-15 minutes, or until the salmon is cooked through and flakes easily with a fork.

11. Carefully open the foil packets (watch out for steam) and transfer the salmon fillets to serving plates.

12. Garnish with additional fresh dill and lemon slices if desired. Serve the lemon dill salmon hot, with your favorite side dishes.

54. Grilled chicken souvlaki skewers

Ingredients:
- 1.5 lbs boneless, skinless chicken breasts or thighs, cut into bite-sized pieces
- 1/4 cup olive oil
- 3 tablespoons lemon juice
- 2 cloves garlic, minced
- 1 teaspoon dried oregano
- 1 teaspoon dried thyme
- 1 teaspoon dried rosemary
- Salt and pepper to taste
- Wooden or metal skewers

Instructions:

1. If using wooden skewers, soak them in water for at least 30 minutes to prevent them from burning on the grill.

2. In a bowl, combine the olive oil, lemon juice, minced garlic, dried oregano, dried thyme, dried rosemary, salt, and pepper. Mix well to combine.

3. Add the chicken pieces to the marinade and toss to coat evenly. Cover the bowl and refrigerate for at least 30 minutes, or up to 2 hours, to allow the flavors to meld.

4. Preheat your grill to medium-high heat.

5. Thread the marinated chicken pieces onto the skewers, leaving a little space between each piece.

6. Place the chicken skewers on the preheated grill and cook for 6-8 minutes per side, or until the chicken is cooked through and nicely charred on the outside.

7. Once the chicken is cooked through, remove the skewers from the grill and let them rest for a few minutes.

8. Serve the grilled chicken souvlaki skewers hot, garnished with fresh herbs like parsley or oregano, and accompanied by tzatziki sauce, pita bread, and your favorite Greek sides.

Enjoy your delicious and aromatic grilled chicken souvlaki skewers!

55. Shrimp fajitas

Ingredients:
- 1 lb large shrimp, peeled and deveined
- 2 bell peppers (any color), sliced
- 1 onion, sliced
- 2 cloves garlic, minced
- 2 tablespoons olive oil
- 1 tablespoon chili powder
- 1 teaspoon ground cumin
- 1 teaspoon paprika
- 1/2 teaspoon garlic powder
- 1/2 teaspoon onion powder
- Salt and pepper to taste
- Flour or corn tortillas, for serving
- Optional toppings: salsa, sour cream, guacamole, shredded cheese, chopped cilantro, lime wedges

Instructions:
1. In a small bowl, mix together the chili powder, ground cumin, paprika, garlic powder, onion powder, salt, and pepper.

2. In a large skillet or cast-iron pan, heat the olive oil over medium-high heat.

3. Add the sliced bell peppers and onion to the skillet and cook, stirring occasionally, until they begin to soften, about 5 minutes.

4. Add the minced garlic to the skillet and cook for another 1-2 minutes until fragrant.

5. Push the vegetables to one side of the skillet and add the shrimp to the other side. Sprinkle the seasoning mixture over the shrimp.

6. Cook the shrimp for 2-3 minutes on each side, or until they are pink and opaque.

7. Once the shrimp is cooked through and the vegetables are tender, remove the skillet from the heat.

8. Warm the tortillas according to package instructions.

9. Serve the shrimp and vegetable mixture in warm tortillas, and top with your favorite toppings such as salsa, sour cream, guacamole, shredded cheese, chopped cilantro, and lime wedges. Roll up the tortillas and enjoy your delicious shrimp fajitas!

56. Tuna cakes with avocado salsa

Ingredients:
For the Tuna Cakes:
- 2 cans (5 oz each) tuna, drained
- 1/2 cup breadcrumbs
- 1/4 cup mayonnaise
- 2 green onions, finely chopped
- 1 tablespoon Dijon mustard
- 1 tablespoon lemon juice
- 1 teaspoon Old Bay seasoning (or your favorite seafood seasoning)
- Salt and pepper to taste
- 2 tablespoons olive oil (for frying)

For the Avocado Salsa:
- 2 ripe avocados, diced
- 1 tomato, diced
- 1/4 cup red onion, finely chopped
- 1/4 cup fresh cilantro, chopped
- 1 jalapeño, seeded and minced (optional)
- 1 tablespoon lime juice
- Salt and pepper to taste

Instructions:
1. In a large bowl, combine the drained tuna, breadcrumbs, mayonnaise, chopped green onions, Dijon mustard, lemon juice, Old Bay seasoning, salt, and pepper. Mix until well combined.

2. Form the tuna mixture into patties, using about 1/4 cup of mixture for each patty.

3. Heat the olive oil in a skillet over medium heat. Once hot, add the tuna cakes to the skillet and cook for 3-4 minutes on each side, or until golden brown and heated through.

4. While the tuna cakes are cooking, prepare the avocado salsa. In a medium bowl, combine the diced avocados, tomato, red onion, chopped cilantro, jalapeño (if using), lime juice, salt, and pepper. Gently toss to combine.

5. Once the tuna cakes are cooked, remove them from the skillet and transfer to a plate lined with paper towels to drain any excess oil.

6. Serve the tuna cakes hot, topped with the avocado salsa. Enjoy your flavorful and satisfying tuna cakes with avocado salsa!

57. Black bean and veggie quesadillas

Ingredients:
- 1 can (15 oz) black beans, drained and rinsed
- 1 bell pepper, diced
- 1 onion, diced
- 1 cup corn kernels (fresh, frozen, or canned)
- 1 teaspoon ground cumin
- 1/2 teaspoon chili powder
- Salt and pepper to taste
- 4 large flour tortillas
- 2 cups shredded cheese (such as cheddar, Monterey Jack, or a Mexican blend)
- Olive oil or cooking spray, for cooking
- Optional toppings: salsa, guacamole, sour cream, chopped cilantro, lime wedges

Instructions:

1. In a large skillet, heat a drizzle of olive oil over medium heat. Add the diced bell pepper and onion, and cook until softened, about 5 minutes.

2. Add the corn kernels to the skillet, along with the drained and rinsed black beans, ground cumin, chili powder, salt, and pepper. Stir well to combine, and cook for another 2-3 minutes until heated through. Remove from heat.

3. Heat a separate large skillet or griddle over medium heat. Lightly grease the skillet with olive oil or cooking spray.

4. Place one flour tortilla in the skillet. Spread a layer of the black bean and veggie mixture evenly over half of the tortilla.

5. Sprinkle a generous amount of shredded cheese over the black bean mixture.

6. Fold the empty half of the tortilla over the filling to create a half-moon shape.

7. Cook the quesadilla for 2-3 minutes on each side, or until golden brown and crispy, and the cheese is melted.

8. Remove the cooked quesadilla from the skillet and transfer to a cutting board. Let it cool for a minute, then use a sharp knife to cut it into wedges. Repeat the process with the remaining tortillas and filling ingredients.

9. Serve the black bean and veggie quesadillas hot, with your favorite toppings such as salsa, guacamole, sour cream, chopped cilantro, and lime wedges. Enjoy your delicious and flavorful black bean and veggie quesadillas!

These quesadillas are versatile, so feel free to customize them with your favorite veggies and toppings. They're perfect for a quick lunch or dinner, and you can even make them ahead of time and reheat them for a convenient meal option.

58. Chickpea and vegetable curry

Ingredients:
- 1 tablespoon oil
(such as olive oil or coconut oil)
- 1 onion, finely chopped
- 3 cloves garlic, minced
- 1 tablespoon grated fresh ginger
- 2 teaspoons curry powder
- 1 teaspoon ground cumin
- 1/2 teaspoon ground turmeric
- 1/2 teaspoon ground coriander
- 1/4 teaspoon cayenne pepper (optional, for heat)
- 1 can (14 oz) diced tomatoes
- 1 can (14 oz) coconut milk
- 2 cups cooked chickpeas (or 1 can, drained and rinsed)
- 2 cups mixed vegetables (such as bell peppers, carrots, peas, and spinach)
- Salt and pepper to taste
- Fresh cilantro, chopped, for garnish (optional)
- Cooked rice or naan bread, for serving

Instructions:

1. Heat the oil in a large skillet or pot over medium heat. Add the chopped onion and cook until softened, about 5 minutes.

2. Add the minced garlic and grated ginger to the skillet, and cook for another 1-2 minutes until fragrant.

3. Stir in the curry powder, ground cumin, ground turmeric, ground coriander, and cayenne pepper (if using). Cook for 1 minute, stirring constantly, until the spices are fragrant.

4. Add the diced tomatoes (with their juices) to the skillet, and simmer for 5 minutes, stirring occasionally.

5. Pour in the coconut milk and stir to combine. Bring the mixture to a simmer.

6. Add the cooked chickpeas and mixed vegetables to the skillet. Stir well to coat the vegetables and chickpeas in the curry sauce.

7. Cover the skillet and let the curry simmer for 10-15 minutes, or until the vegetables are tender and the flavors have melded together.

8. Season the curry with salt and pepper to taste.

9. Serve the chickpea and vegetable curry hot, garnished with fresh cilantro if desired. Serve with cooked rice or naan bread on the side. Enjoy your delicious and comforting chickpea and vegetable curry!

This curry is versatile, so feel free to customize it with your favorite vegetables and adjust the spices to suit your taste. It's a great way to enjoy a nutritious and satisfying meal packed with protein and flavor.

59. Pork tenderloin with apple chutney

Ingredients:
For the Pork Tenderloin:
- 1 pork tenderloin (about 1 lb)
- Salt and pepper to taste
- 1 tablespoon olive oil

For the Apple Chutney:
- 2 apples, peeled, cored, and diced
- 1/2 cup apple cider vinegar
- 1/4 cup brown sugar
- 1/4 cup raisins or dried cranberries
- 1/2 teaspoon ground cinnamon
- 1/4 teaspoon ground ginger
- Pinch of salt

Instructions:
1. Preheat your oven to 400°F (200°C).

2. Season the pork tenderloin generously with salt and pepper on all sides.

3. Heat the olive oil in an ovenproof skillet over medium-high heat. Once hot, add the pork tenderloin to the skillet and sear it on all sides until browned, about 2-3 minutes per side.

4. Transfer the skillet to the preheated oven and roast the pork tenderloin for 15-20 minutes, or until it reaches an internal temperature of 145°F (63°C) for medium-rare or 160°F (71°C) for medium.

5. While the pork tenderloin is roasting, prepare the apple chutney. In a medium saucepan, combine the diced apples, apple cider vinegar, brown sugar, raisins or dried cranberries, ground cinnamon, ground ginger, and a pinch of salt.

6. Bring the mixture to a simmer over medium heat. Reduce the heat to low and let the chutney simmer gently for 15-20 minutes, stirring occasionally, until the apples are soft and the mixture has thickened slightly.

7. Once the pork tenderloin is done roasting, remove it from the oven and let it rest for a few minutes before slicing.

8. Slice the pork tenderloin into medallions and serve it hot with the apple chutney spooned over the top. Enjoy your delicious pork tenderloin with apple chutney!

60. Grilled turkey burgers

Ingredients:
- 1 lb ground turkey (preferably lean)
- 1/4 cup breadcrumbs
- 1/4 cup grated Parmesan cheese
- 1/4 cup finely chopped onion
- 2 cloves garlic, minced
- 1 tablespoon Worcestershire sauce
- 1 teaspoon dried oregano
- 1 teaspoon dried basil
- 1/2 teaspoon salt
- 1/4 teaspoon black pepper
- Olive oil or cooking spray, for grilling
- Hamburger buns and your favorite toppings, for serving

Instructions:
1. Preheat your grill to medium-high heat.

2. In a large bowl, combine the ground turkey, breadcrumbs, grated Parmesan cheese, finely chopped onion, minced garlic, Worcestershire sauce, dried oregano, dried basil, salt, and black pepper. Mix until well combined.

3. Divide the turkey mixture into 4 equal portions and shape each portion into a burger patty.

4. Lightly oil the grill grates with olive oil or cooking spray to prevent sticking.

5. Place the turkey burger patties on the preheated grill and cook for 5-6 minutes per side, or until they are cooked through and reach an internal temperature of 165°F (74°C).

6. While the turkey burgers are cooking, toast the hamburger buns on the grill for a minute or two, if desired.

7. Once the turkey burgers are done cooking, remove them from the grill and let them rest for a few minutes.

8. Assemble the grilled turkey burgers on the toasted hamburger buns and top with your favorite toppings such as lettuce, tomato, onion, avocado, cheese, ketchup, mustard, or mayonnaise. Serve the grilled turkey burgers hot and enjoy!

These grilled turkey burgers are juicy, flavorful, and a healthier option for your next barbecue or weeknight dinner. Feel free to customize them with your favorite toppings

61. Brown rice pilaf with mushrooms

Ingredients:
- 1 cup brown rice
- 2 cups vegetable or chicken broth
- 1 tablespoon olive oil or butter
- 1 small onion, finely chopped
- 2 cloves garlic, minced
- 8 oz mushrooms (such as cremini or button), sliced
- 1/4 teaspoon dried thyme
- 1/4 teaspoon dried rosemary
- Salt and pepper to taste
- 2 tablespoons chopped fresh parsley (optional), for garnish

Instructions:
1. Rinse the brown rice under cold water until the water runs clear. This helps remove excess starch and prevents the rice from becoming sticky.

2. In a medium saucepan, heat the olive oil or butter over medium heat. Add the chopped onion and cook until softened, about 5 minutes.

3. Add the minced garlic to the saucepan and cook for another 1-2 minutes until fragrant.

4. Stir in the sliced mushrooms and cook for 5-7 minutes, or until the mushrooms have released their moisture and are lightly browned.

5. Add the brown rice to the saucepan and stir to coat the rice in the oil and vegetables.

6. Pour in the vegetable or chicken broth and add the dried thyme and rosemary. Season with salt and pepper to taste.

7. Bring the mixture to a boil, then reduce the heat to low. Cover the saucepan with a lid and let the rice simmer for 40-45 minutes, or until the rice is tender and has absorbed all the liquid.

8. Once the rice is cooked, remove the saucepan from the heat and let it sit, covered, for 5 minutes to steam.

9. Fluff the rice pilaf with a fork and transfer it to a serving dish. Garnish the brown rice pilaf with chopped fresh parsley, if desired, and serve hot.

Enjoy your flavorful and aromatic brown rice pilaf with mushrooms as a side dish to complement your meal!

62. Roasted sweet potato wedges

Ingredients:
- 2 large sweet potatoes
- 2 tablespoons olive oil
- 1 teaspoon smoked paprika
- 1/2 teaspoon garlic powder
- 1/2 teaspoon onion powder
- 1/2 teaspoon dried thyme
- Salt and pepper to taste
- Optional: chopped fresh parsley or cilantro for garnish

Instructions:
1. Preheat your oven to 425°F (220°C) and line a baking sheet with parchment paper or aluminum foil for easy cleanup.

2. Scrub the sweet potatoes clean and pat them dry with a paper towel. Cut each sweet potato into wedges, about 1/2 inch thick.

3. In a large bowl, toss the sweet potato wedges with olive oil until evenly coated.

4. In a small bowl, mix together the smoked paprika, garlic powder, onion powder, dried thyme, salt, and pepper.

5. Sprinkle the spice mixture over the sweet potato wedges and toss to coat evenly.

6. Arrange the seasoned sweet potato wedges in a single layer on the prepared baking sheet, making sure they are not crowded.

7. Roast the sweet potato wedges in the preheated oven for 20-25 minutes, flipping halfway through, or until they are tender and lightly browned on the edges.

8. Once the sweet potato wedges are done roasting, remove them from the oven and transfer them to a serving dish.

9. Garnish the roasted sweet potato wedges with chopped fresh parsley or cilantro, if desired, and serve hot.

Enjoy your flavorful and crispy roasted sweet potato wedges as a tasty side dish to accompany your meal!

63. Sauteed spinach with garlic

Ingredients:
- 1 tablespoon olive oil
- 2 cloves garlic, minced
- 1 lb fresh spinach, washed and stems removed
- Salt and pepper to taste
- Optional: red pepper flakes, lemon zest

Instructions:
1. Heat the olive oil in a large skillet over medium heat.

2. Add the minced garlic to the skillet and sauté for about 30 seconds, or until fragrant.

3. Add the fresh spinach to the skillet in batches, allowing each batch to wilt slightly before adding more. Use tongs to toss the spinach as it cooks.

4. Continue cooking and tossing the spinach until all the leaves are wilted and tender, about 3-5 minutes.

5. Season the sautéed spinach with salt and pepper to taste. You can also add a pinch of red pepper flakes for heat or a sprinkle of lemon zest for brightness, if desired.

6. Once the spinach is cooked to your liking, remove the skillet from the heat.

7. Transfer the sautéed spinach to a serving dish and serve hot.

Enjoy your flavorful and nutritious sautéed spinach with garlic as a delicious side dish!

64. Whole wheat couscous salad

Ingredients:
- 1 cup whole wheat couscous
- 1 1/4 cups water or vegetable broth
- 1 tablespoon olive oil
- 1 tablespoon lemon juice
- 1 teaspoon Dijon mustard
- Salt and pepper to taste
- 1 cucumber, diced
- 1 bell pepper (any color), diced
- 1 cup cherry tomatoes, halved
- 1/4 cup red onion, finely chopped
- 1/4 cup fresh parsley, chopped
- Optional: crumbled feta cheese, olives, chickpeas, avocado

Instructions:

1. In a medium saucepan, bring the water or vegetable broth to a boil.

2. Stir in the whole wheat couscous, cover the saucepan, and remove it from the heat. Let it sit for 5 minutes to allow the couscous to absorb the liquid.

3. Fluff the cooked couscous with a fork and transfer it to a large mixing bowl. Let it cool slightly.

4. In a small bowl, whisk together the olive oil, lemon juice, Dijon mustard, salt, and pepper to make the dressing.

5. Pour the dressing over the cooked couscous and toss to coat evenly.

6. Add the diced cucumber, bell pepper, cherry tomatoes, red onion, and chopped parsley to the bowl with the couscous. Toss gently to combine.

7. If desired, add any optional ingredients such as crumbled feta cheese, olives, chickpeas, or avocado.

8. Taste and adjust the seasoning if needed, adding more salt, pepper, or lemon juice as desired.

9. Cover the couscous salad and refrigerate for at least 30 minutes to allow the flavors to meld together.

10. Serve the whole wheat couscous salad chilled or at room temperature, garnished with additional fresh herbs if desired.

Enjoy your flavorful and nutritious whole wheat couscous salad! It's a versatile dish that you can customize with your favorite vegetables and add-ins.

65. Quinoa with dried cranberries and pecans

Ingredients:
- 1 cup quinoa
- 2 cups water or vegetable broth
- 1/2 cup dried cranberries
- 1/2 cup pecans, chopped
- 2 tablespoons olive oil
- 2 tablespoons lemon juice
- 1 tablespoon honey or maple syrup
- Salt and pepper to taste
- Optional: chopped fresh parsley or mint for garnish

Instructions:

1. Rinse the quinoa under cold water in a fine-mesh sieve until the water runs clear.

2. In a medium saucepan, combine the rinsed quinoa and water or vegetable broth. Bring to a boil over medium-high heat.

3. Once boiling, reduce the heat to low, cover, and simmer for 15-20 minutes, or until the quinoa is cooked and the liquid is absorbed.

4. Remove the saucepan from the heat and let the quinoa sit, covered, for 5 minutes. Then, fluff the quinoa with a fork and transfer it to a large mixing bowl to cool slightly.

5. In a small bowl, whisk together the olive oil, lemon juice, honey or maple syrup, salt, and pepper to make the dressing.

6. Pour the dressing over the cooked quinoa and toss to coat evenly.

7. Add the dried cranberries and chopped pecans to the bowl with the quinoa and toss gently to combine.

8. Taste and adjust the seasoning if needed, adding more salt, pepper, or lemon juice as desired.

9. If desired, garnish the quinoa salad with chopped fresh parsley or mint for a burst of freshness.

10. Serve the quinoa with dried cranberries and pecans warm, at room temperature, or chilled, depending on your preference.

Enjoy your flavorful and nutritious quinoa salad with dried cranberries and pecans! It's a perfect side dish for any meal or a light and satisfying lunch on its own.

66. Apple with almond butter

Ingredients:
- 1 apple (any variety), cored and sliced
- Almond butter (or your favorite nut or seed butter)

Instructions:

1. Wash the apple thoroughly under cold water and pat it dry with a paper towel.

2. Core the apple and slice it into wedges or rounds, depending on your preference. You can also leave the apple whole and slice it into thick rounds or use a melon baller to remove the core and create apple "rings."

3. Spread a generous amount of almond butter onto each apple slice or serve it on the side for dipping.

4. Enjoy your apple slices with almond butter as a nutritious and satisfying snack!

You can customize this snack by adding toppings such as sliced bananas, berries, granola, chia seeds, or a sprinkle of cinnamon for extra flavor and texture. It's a great option for a quick snack, breakfast, or pre-workout fuel that will keep you feeling full and energized.

67. Cottage cheese with fruit

Ingredients:

- Cottage cheese (any variety, such as full-fat, low-fat, or fat-free)
- Fresh fruit (such as berries, sliced peaches, pineapple chunks, or grapes)
- Optional toppings: honey, maple syrup, chopped nuts, granola, cinnamon

Instructions:

1. Choose your favorite variety of cottage cheese and scoop it into a serving bowl or plate.

2. Wash and prepare your fresh fruit by rinsing berries, slicing peaches, or chopping pineapple or other fruits into bite-sized pieces.

3. Arrange the fresh fruit on top of the cottage cheese, either in a neat pattern or scattered across the surface.

4. If desired, drizzle a small amount of honey or maple syrup over the cottage cheese and fruit for added sweetness.

5. Optional: sprinkle chopped nuts, granola, or a pinch of cinnamon over the top for extra flavor and texture.

6. Serve your cottage cheese with fruit immediately and enjoy it as a nutritious snack or breakfast option.

Cottage cheese with fruit is versatile and can be customized with your favorite fruits and toppings to suit your taste preferences. It's a delicious and satisfying option that provides a balance of protein, carbohydrates, and healthy fats to keep you feeling full and energized.

68. Hard boiled eggs

Ingredients:

- Eggs (as many as you'd like)

Instructions:

1. Place the eggs in a single layer in a saucepan or pot. Make sure they are not crowded, as they need space to cook evenly.

2. Fill the saucepan or pot with enough cold water to cover the eggs by about an inch.

3. Place the saucepan or pot on the stove over high heat and bring the water to a rolling boil.

4. Once the water is boiling, cover the saucepan or pot with a lid and remove it from the heat.

5. Let the eggs sit in the hot water, covered, for 10-12 minutes for medium-sized eggs (adjust cooking time slightly for smaller or larger eggs).

6. While the eggs are cooking, prepare a bowl of ice water.

7. After the eggs have finished cooking, immediately transfer them to the bowl of ice water using a slotted spoon or tongs. This will stop the cooking process and help prevent the eggs from overcooking.

8. Let the eggs cool in the ice water for at least 5 minutes.

9. Once cooled, remove the eggs from the ice water and gently tap them on a hard surface to crack the shells.

10. Peel the shells off the eggs under cool running water, starting from the wider end where the air pocket is located.

11. Once peeled, pat the eggs dry with a paper towel and serve them immediately, or store them in the refrigerator for later use.

Enjoy your perfectly cooked hard-boiled eggs as a snack, salad topping, or protein-packed addition to your meals!

69. Trail mix with whole grain cereal

Ingredients:

- 1 cup whole grain cereal (such as whole grain flakes, puffs, or squares)
- 1/2 cup nuts (such as almonds, walnuts, or cashews)
- 1/2 cup dried fruit (such as raisins, cranberries, or apricots)
- 1/4 cup seeds (such as pumpkin seeds or sunflower seeds)
- Optional: chocolate chips, coconut flakes, pretzel pieces, or other favorite mix-ins

Instructions:

1. In a large mixing bowl, combine the whole grain cereal, nuts, dried fruit, and seeds.

2. If using any optional mix-ins such as chocolate chips, coconut flakes, or pretzel pieces, add them to the bowl as well.

3. Toss the ingredients together until evenly distributed.

4. Transfer the trail mix to an airtight container or portion it out into individual snack bags for easy grab-and-go convenience.

5. Enjoy your homemade trail mix with whole grain cereal as a nutritious and satisfying snack anytime you need a boost of energy!

This trail mix is customizable, so feel free to experiment with different combinations of nuts, dried fruit, seeds, and mix-ins to suit your taste preferences. It's a great way to incorporate whole grains into your snack routine while enjoying a delicious and satisfying treat.

70. Cucumber slices with Everything Bagel seasoning

Ingredients:
- 1 large cucumber
- Everything Bagel seasoning (store-bought or homemade)
- Optional: cream cheese or Greek yogurt for dipping

Instructions:
1. Wash the cucumber thoroughly under cold water and pat it dry with a paper towel.

2. Slice the cucumber into thin rounds using a sharp knife or a mandoline slicer. Alternatively, you can slice the cucumber into spears or sticks if preferred.

3. Arrange the cucumber slices on a serving platter or plate in a single layer.

4. Sprinkle the Everything Bagel seasoning generously over the cucumber slices, making sure each slice is well coated.

5. If desired, serve the cucumber slices with a side of cream cheese or Greek yogurt for dipping.

6. Enjoy your cucumber slices with Everything Bagel seasoning as a refreshing and flavorful snack or appetizer!

These cucumber slices are light, crunchy, and bursting with savory flavor from the Everything Bagel seasoning. They're perfect for serving at parties, picnics, or as a healthy snack any time of the day.

71. Steel cut oatmeal with blueberries and walnuts

Ingredients:
- 1 cup steel-cut oats
- 3 cups water
- Pinch of salt
- 1 cup fresh or frozen blueberries
- 1/4 cup chopped walnuts
- Optional toppings: honey, maple syrup, cinnamon, milk or yogurt

Instructions:
1. In a medium saucepan, bring the water to a boil over high heat.

2. Once the water is boiling, stir in the steel-cut oats and a pinch of salt.

3. Reduce the heat to low and simmer the oats, uncovered, for 20-25 minutes, stirring occasionally, until they are tender and creamy.

4. While the oats are cooking, rinse the blueberries under cold water if using fresh ones. If using frozen blueberries, you can thaw them in the microwave or let them thaw at room temperature.

5. Once the oats are cooked to your desired consistency, remove the saucepan from the heat.

6. Divide the cooked steel-cut oats into serving bowls.

7. Top the oatmeal with the fresh or thawed blueberries and chopped walnuts.

8. If desired, drizzle a small amount of honey or maple syrup over the oatmeal for added sweetness.

9. Optional: sprinkle a pinch of cinnamon over the oatmeal for extra flavor.

10. Serve the steel-cut oatmeal with blueberries and walnuts hot, along with milk or yogurt on the side if desired.

11. Enjoy your nutritious and delicious breakfast of steel-cut oatmeal with blueberries and walnuts!

This hearty breakfast will keep you feeling full and satisfied until lunchtime, and it's a great way to start your day on a healthy note. Feel free to customize the oatmeal with your favorite toppings and add-ins to suit your taste preferences.

72. Veggie frittata

Ingredients:
- 8 large eggs
- 1/4 cup milk or half-and-half
- Salt and pepper to taste
- 1 tablespoon olive oil
- 1 small onion, diced
- 1 bell pepper, diced
- 1 cup sliced mushrooms
- 1 cup baby spinach leaves
- 1/2 cup cherry tomatoes, halved
- 1/2 cup shredded cheese (such as cheddar, mozzarella, or feta)
- Optional: chopped fresh herbs (such as parsley, basil, or chives) for garnish

Instructions:
1. Preheat your oven to 350°F (175°C).

2. In a large mixing bowl, whisk together the eggs, milk or half-and-half, salt, and pepper until well combined. Set aside.

3. Heat the olive oil in a large ovenproof skillet over medium heat.

4. Add the diced onion and bell pepper to the skillet and cook until softened, about 5 minutes.

5. Add the sliced mushrooms to the skillet and cook for another 3-4 minutes, until they are tender and any excess moisture has evaporated.

6. Stir in the baby spinach leaves and cook until wilted, about 1-2 minutes.

7. Pour the egg mixture into the skillet, making sure the veggies are evenly distributed.

8. Arrange the halved cherry tomatoes on top of the egg mixture, cut side up.

9. Sprinkle the shredded cheese evenly over the top of the frittata.

10. Transfer the skillet to the preheated oven and bake the frittata for 20-25 minutes, or until the eggs are set in the center and the top is golden brown.

11. Once the frittata is done baking, remove it from the oven and let it cool for a few minutes. Slice the veggie frittata into wedges or squares, garnish with chopped fresh herbs if desired, and serve hot.

Enjoy your flavorful and nutritious veggie frittata as a delicious meal any time of day! It's a great way to use up leftover vegetables and can be customized with your favorite veggies and cheese.

73. Whole wheat banana bread

Ingredients:
- 3 ripe bananas, mashed
- 1/3 cup melted coconut oil or vegetable oil
- 1/2 cup honey or maple syrup
- 2 eggs
- 1 teaspoon vanilla extract
- 1 teaspoon baking soda
- 1/4 teaspoon salt
- 1/2 teaspoon ground cinnamon
- 1 3/4 cups whole wheat flour
- Optional: 1/2 cup chopped nuts or chocolate chips for extra flavor

Instructions:
1. Preheat your oven to 325°F (165°C). Grease a 9x5-inch loaf pan or line it with parchment paper for easy removal.

2. In a large mixing bowl, combine the mashed bananas, melted coconut oil or vegetable oil, honey or maple syrup, eggs, and vanilla extract. Mix until well combined.

3. Add the baking soda, salt, and ground cinnamon to the wet ingredients and stir until evenly incorporated.

4. Gradually add the whole wheat flour to the wet ingredients, mixing until just combined. Be careful not to overmix.

5. If using, fold in the chopped nuts or chocolate chips until evenly distributed throughout the batter.

6. Pour the batter into the prepared loaf pan and spread it out evenly with a spatula.

7. Bake the whole wheat banana bread in the preheated oven for 50-60 minutes, or until a toothpick inserted into the center comes out clean.

8. Once done, remove the banana bread from the oven and let it cool in the pan for 10 minutes.

9. After 10 minutes, carefully transfer the banana bread to a wire rack to cool completely.

10. Once cooled, slice the whole wheat banana bread into thick slices and serve.

74. Greek yogurt with fresh berries and chia seeds

Ingredients:

- Greek yogurt (plain or flavored, whichever you prefer)
- Fresh berries (such as strawberries, blueberries, raspberries, or blackberries)
- Chia seeds

Instructions:

1. Spoon the desired amount of Greek yogurt into a serving bowl or glass.

2. Wash the fresh berries under cold water and pat them dry with a paper towel. Slice any larger berries into smaller pieces if desired.

3. Arrange the fresh berries on top of the Greek yogurt.

4. Sprinkle chia seeds over the yogurt and berries, to taste. Chia seeds add texture and are rich in fiber, omega-3 fatty acids, and protein.

5. Optional: drizzle a small amount of honey or maple syrup over the yogurt and berries for added sweetness, if desired.

6. Stir the yogurt, berries, and chia seeds together gently to combine, or leave them layered for a beautiful presentation.

7. Serve the Greek yogurt with fresh berries and chia seeds immediately and enjoy it as a nutritious and delicious snack or breakfast option!

This simple and customizable dish is quick to prepare and can be enjoyed any time of day. Feel free to experiment with different types of berries, flavored Greek yogurt, or additional toppings such as granola or chopped nuts to suit your taste preferences.

75. Avocado toast with tomato and arugula

Ingredients:
- 1 ripe avocado
- 2 slices of whole grain bread, toasted
- 1 medium tomato, sliced
- Handful of fresh arugula
- Salt and pepper to taste
- Optional toppings: lemon juice, red pepper flakes, balsamic glaze, sesame seeds

Instructions:

1. Cut the ripe avocado in half and remove the pit. Scoop the avocado flesh into a small bowl and mash it with a fork until smooth and creamy.

2. Season the mashed avocado with salt and pepper to taste. If desired, you can also add a squeeze of lemon juice for extra flavor.

3. Toast the slices of whole grain bread until golden brown and crispy.

4. Spread the mashed avocado evenly onto the toasted bread slices.

5. Top the avocado toast with sliced tomato and a handful of fresh arugula.

6. If desired, drizzle a small amount of balsamic glaze over the avocado toast for added flavor and sweetness.

7. Sprinkle red pepper flakes or sesame seeds over the avocado toast for extra heat or crunch, if desired.

8. Serve the avocado toast with tomato and arugula immediately and enjoy it as a nutritious and delicious breakfast or snack!

This avocado toast is quick and easy to make, and it's a great way to start your day on a healthy note. Feel free to customize it with your favorite toppings and seasonings to suit your taste preferences.

76. Tahini sauce for falafel or veggies

Ingredients:
- 1/2 cup tahini (sesame seed paste)
- 1/4 cup water
- 2 tablespoons lemon juice
- 1 clove garlic, minced
- Salt to taste
- Optional: chopped fresh parsley or cilantro for garnish

Instructions:
1. In a small mixing bowl, whisk together the tahini, water, lemon juice, minced garlic, and a pinch of salt until smooth and creamy. The mixture may thicken initially, but keep whisking until it reaches a smooth consistency.

2. Taste the tahini sauce and adjust the seasoning, adding more lemon juice or salt if needed to suit your taste preferences.

3. If the tahini sauce is too thick, you can add a little more water, one tablespoon at a time, until you reach the desired consistency. If it's too thin, you can add a little more tahini.

4. Once the tahini sauce is smooth and creamy and seasoned to your liking, transfer it to a serving bowl.

5. Optional: garnish the tahini sauce with chopped fresh parsley or cilantro for a pop of color and freshness.

6. Serve the tahini sauce alongside falafel, grilled veggies, roasted vegetables, or use it as a dressing for salads or grain bowls.

7. Store any leftover tahini sauce in an airtight container in the refrigerator for up to one week. Stir well before using, as it may separate upon standing.

Enjoy your homemade tahini sauce as a delicious and versatile condiment for a variety of dishes!

77. Mango salsa

Ingredients:
- 2 ripe mangos, diced
- 1/2 red bell pepper, diced
- 1/4 cup red onion, finely chopped
- 1 jalapeño pepper, seeded and minced
- 1/4 cup fresh cilantro, chopped
- Juice of 1 lime
- Salt and pepper to taste

Instructions:

1. In a medium mixing bowl, combine the diced mangos, red bell pepper, red onion, minced jalapeño pepper, and chopped cilantro.

2. Squeeze the juice of one lime over the mango mixture and toss gently to combine.

3. Season the mango salsa with salt and pepper to taste, adjusting the seasoning as needed.

4. Once the salsa is well mixed and seasoned, cover the bowl with plastic wrap and refrigerate for at least 30 minutes to allow the flavors to meld together.

5. After chilling, taste the mango salsa and adjust the seasoning if needed with additional lime juice, salt, or pepper.

6. Serve the mango salsa immediately as a topping for grilled fish, chicken, or tacos, or as a dip with tortilla chips.

7. Store any leftover mango salsa in an airtight container in the refrigerator for up to two days. Stir well before serving, as the juices may separate upon standing.

Enjoy your homemade mango salsa as a delicious and refreshing accompaniment to your favorite dishes!

78. Apple cider vinaigrette

Ingredients:
- 1/4 cup apple cider vinegar
- 2 tablespoons honey or maple syrup
- 1 tablespoon Dijon mustard
- 1/2 cup extra-virgin olive oil
- Salt and pepper to taste

Instructions:

1. In a small mixing bowl or jar, whisk together the apple cider vinegar, honey or maple syrup, and Dijon mustard until well combined.

2. Slowly drizzle in the extra-virgin olive oil while whisking continuously, until the dressing is emulsified and smooth.

3. Season the apple cider vinaigrette with salt and pepper to taste, adjusting the seasoning as needed.

4. Once the vinaigrette is well mixed and seasoned, transfer it to an airtight container or dressing bottle.

5. Store the apple cider vinaigrette in the refrigerator for up to one week.

6. Before using, shake or stir the dressing well to re-emulsify any separated ingredients.

7. Serve the apple cider vinaigrette drizzled over your favorite salads, or use it as a marinade for grilled vegetables or proteins.

Enjoy your homemade apple cider vinaigrette as a flavorful and refreshing addition to your meals! Adjust the sweetness and acidity levels to suit your taste preferences.

79. Peanut dressing for salads or veggie dip

Ingredients:
- 1/4 cup peanut butter (smooth or crunchy)
- 2 tablespoons soy sauce or tamari
- 2 tablespoons rice vinegar
- 1 tablespoon honey or maple syrup
- 1 clove garlic, minced
- 1 teaspoon grated fresh ginger
- 1-2 tablespoons water (to adjust consistency)
- Optional: sriracha or chili garlic sauce for heat
- Optional: chopped peanuts or sesame seeds for garnish

Instructions:

1. In a small mixing bowl, combine the peanut butter, soy sauce or tamari, rice vinegar, honey or maple syrup, minced garlic, and grated fresh ginger.

2. Whisk the ingredients together until smooth and well combined. If the dressing is too thick, add water, one tablespoon at a time, until you reach your desired consistency.

3. Taste the peanut dressing and adjust the seasoning as needed. You can add more soy sauce for saltiness, honey or maple syrup for sweetness, or grated ginger for freshness.

4. For a spicy kick, you can add a dash of sriracha or chili garlic sauce to the dressing, to taste.

5. Once the peanut dressing is well mixed and seasoned to your liking, transfer it to a serving bowl or jar.

6. Optional: garnish the peanut dressing with chopped peanuts or sesame seeds for added texture and flavor.

7. Serve the peanut dressing with your favorite salads or as a dip for raw vegetables like carrot sticks, cucumber slices, or bell pepper strips.

8. Store any leftover peanut dressing in an airtight container in the refrigerator for up to one week. Stir well before using, as the ingredients may separate upon standing.

Enjoy your homemade peanut dressing as a creamy and flavorful addition to your salads or as a tasty dip for veggies! Adjust the sweetness, saltiness, and spiciness levels to suit your taste preferences.

80. Chimichurri sauce for meats or veggies

Ingredients:
- 1 cup fresh parsley leaves, packed
- 1/4 cup fresh cilantro leaves, packed
- 3 cloves garlic, minced
- 2 tablespoons red wine vinegar or apple cider vinegar
- 1/2 teaspoon dried oregano
- 1/2 teaspoon red pepper flakes (adjust to taste)
- 1/2 cup extra-virgin olive oil
- Salt and pepper to taste
- Optional: 1 tablespoon fresh lemon juice

Instructions:

1. In a food processor or blender, combine the fresh parsley, fresh cilantro, minced garlic, red wine vinegar or apple cider vinegar, dried oregano, and red pepper flakes.

2. Pulse the ingredients a few times until they are finely chopped and well combined.

3. While the food processor or blender is running, slowly drizzle in the extra-virgin olive oil until the chimichurri sauce reaches a smooth and pourable consistency.

4. Taste the chimichurri sauce and season with salt and pepper to taste. If desired, add a splash of fresh lemon juice for extra brightness.

5. Once the chimichurri sauce is well mixed and seasoned to your liking, transfer it to a serving bowl or jar.

6. Serve the chimichurri sauce alongside grilled meats such as steak, chicken, or pork, or drizzle it over roasted vegetables or grilled tofu for a burst of flavor.

7. Store any leftover chimichurri sauce in an airtight container in the refrigerator for up to one week. Stir well before using, as the ingredients may separate upon standing.

Enjoy your homemade chimichurri sauce as a zesty and aromatic addition to your favorite dishes! Adjust the seasoning and spiciness levels to suit your taste preferences.

81. Fresh fruit skewers with honey yogurt dip

Ingredients:
For the fruit skewers:
- Assorted fresh fruits (such as strawberries, pineapple chunks, grapes, melon cubes, kiwi slices, and berries)

For the honey yogurt dip:
- 1 cup Greek yogurt
- 2 tablespoons honey (adjust to taste)
- 1 teaspoon vanilla extract (optional)

Instructions:

1. Prepare the fruit by washing it thoroughly under cold water. Pat the fruits dry with a paper towel.

2. Chop the larger fruits (such as melon or pineapple) into bite-sized cubes or chunks, and leave smaller fruits (such as berries) whole or halved.

3. Thread the assorted fruits onto wooden or metal skewers in any pattern you like. Leave a little space at the bottom of each skewer for easy handling.

4. In a small bowl, mix together the Greek yogurt, honey, and vanilla extract (if using) until well combined. Taste the dip and adjust the sweetness by adding more honey if desired.

5. Transfer the honey yogurt dip to a serving bowl.

6. Arrange the fruit skewers on a platter or serving tray alongside the bowl of honey yogurt dip.

7. Serve the fresh fruit skewers with honey yogurt dip as a refreshing and nutritious snack or dessert option.

Enjoy your homemade fresh fruit skewers with honey yogurt dip! It's a colorful and delicious treat that's perfect for parties, picnics, or anytime you're craving something sweet and satisfying.

82. Baked apples with cinnamon

Ingredients:
- 4 large apples (such as Granny Smith or Honeycrisp)
- 2 tablespoons unsalted butter, melted
- 2 tablespoons brown sugar or honey
- 1 teaspoon ground cinnamon
- Optional toppings: chopped nuts, raisins, dried cranberries, or a drizzle of maple syrup

Instructions:

1. Preheat your oven to 375°F (190°C). Grease a baking dish or line it with parchment paper for easy cleanup.

2. Wash the apples thoroughly under cold water and pat them dry with a paper towel.

3. Core each apple using a paring knife or an apple corer, removing the seeds and creating a cavity in the center.

4. In a small bowl, mix together the melted butter, brown sugar or honey, and ground cinnamon until well combined.

5. Place the cored apples in the prepared baking dish, standing them upright.

6. Spoon the butter mixture evenly into the cavities of the apples, making sure to coat the inside of each apple with the cinnamon mixture.

7. Optional: sprinkle chopped nuts, raisins, dried cranberries, or any other desired toppings over the top of each apple.

8. Bake the apples in the preheated oven for 25-30 minutes, or until they are tender and the filling is bubbling.

9. Once done, remove the baked apples from the oven and let them cool slightly before serving.

10. Serve the baked apples warm, either on their own or with a scoop of vanilla ice cream or a dollop of whipped cream.

Enjoy your homemade baked apples with cinnamon as a delicious and comforting dessert! Adjust the sweetness and seasoning to suit your taste preferences.

83. Dark chocolate avocado pudding

Ingredients:
- 2 ripe avocados
- 1/2 cup unsweetened cocoa powder
- 1/4 cup maple syrup or honey (adjust to taste)
- 1 teaspoon vanilla extract
- Pinch of salt
- 1/4 cup almond milk or any milk of your choice (add more if needed for consistency)
- Optional toppings: fresh berries, sliced bananas, chopped nuts, shredded coconut

Instructions:
1. Cut the avocados in half and remove the pits. Scoop out the flesh and place it in a food processor or blender.

2. Add the unsweetened cocoa powder, maple syrup or honey, vanilla extract, salt, and almond milk to the food processor or blender.

3. Blend the ingredients until smooth and creamy, scraping down the sides of the bowl or pitcher as needed to ensure everything is well combined. If the mixture is too thick, you can add more almond milk, a tablespoon at a time, until you reach your desired consistency.

4. Taste the pudding and adjust the sweetness if necessary by adding more maple syrup or honey.

5. Once the pudding is smooth and creamy and seasoned to your liking, transfer it to serving bowls or glasses.

6. Cover the bowls or glasses with plastic wrap and refrigerate the pudding for at least 30 minutes to chill and set.

7. Before serving, garnish the dark chocolate avocado pudding with your favorite toppings, such as fresh berries, sliced bananas, chopped nuts, or shredded coconut.

8. Enjoy your homemade dark chocolate avocado pudding as a delicious and guilt-free dessert!

This rich and creamy pudding is packed with healthy fats from the avocado and antioxidants from the dark chocolate cocoa powder. It's a perfect treat for chocolate lovers looking for a healthier alternative to traditional pudding.

84. Mango chia pudding

Ingredients:

- 1 ripe mango, peeled and diced
- 1 cup unsweetened almond milk or any milk of your choice
- 1/4 cup chia seeds
- 1-2 tablespoons honey or maple syrup (optional, adjust to taste)
- 1/2 teaspoon vanilla extract (optional)
- Optional toppings: diced mango, shredded coconut, chopped nuts, fresh berries

Instructions:

1. In a blender or food processor, puree the diced mango until smooth. If the mango is not very ripe or juicy, you can add a splash of water or almond milk to help it blend.

2. In a mixing bowl, combine the mango puree, unsweetened almond milk, chia seeds, honey or maple syrup (if using), and vanilla extract (if using). Stir well to combine all the ingredients.

3. Cover the bowl and refrigerate the mango chia pudding mixture for at least 2-3 hours, or preferably overnight, to allow the chia seeds to absorb the liquid and thicken the pudding.

4. After chilling, give the mango chia pudding a good stir to redistribute the chia seeds evenly throughout the mixture.

5. Taste the pudding and adjust the sweetness if necessary by adding more honey or maple syrup.

6. Divide the mango chia pudding into serving bowls or glasses.

7. Before serving, garnish the pudding with diced mango, shredded coconut, chopped nuts, or fresh berries, if desired.

8. Enjoy your homemade mango chia pudding as a refreshing and nutritious dessert or snack!

This creamy and flavorful pudding is packed with fiber, omega-3 fatty acids, and antioxidants from the chia seeds and mango. It's a perfect make-ahead option for a quick and healthy breakfast or a satisfying dessert.

85. Peanut butter energy bites

Ingredients:
- 1 cup old-fashioned rolled oats
- 1/2 cup creamy peanut butter
- 1/4 cup honey or maple syrup
- 1/4 cup ground flaxseed or chia seeds
- 1/4 cup mini chocolate chips or chopped nuts (optional)
- 1 teaspoon vanilla extract
- Pinch of salt

Instructions:

1. In a large mixing bowl, combine the old-fashioned rolled oats, creamy peanut butter, honey or maple syrup, ground flaxseed or chia seeds, mini chocolate chips or chopped nuts (if using), vanilla extract, and a pinch of salt.

2. Stir the ingredients together until well combined. The mixture should be thick and sticky.

3. If the mixture seems too dry, you can add a tablespoon or two of water or more peanut butter to help bind everything together.

4. Once the mixture is well mixed and holds together easily, use a small cookie scoop or your hands to shape it into bite-sized balls.

5. Place the peanut butter energy bites on a baking sheet lined with parchment paper or wax paper.

6. Optional: Refrigerate the energy bites for 30 minutes to 1 hour to help them firm up before serving.

7. Store any leftover peanut butter energy bites in an airtight container in the refrigerator for up to one week.

8. Enjoy your homemade peanut butter energy bites as a satisfying and nutritious snack any time of day!

These energy bites are packed with protein, fiber, and healthy fats from the peanut butter and oats, making them a perfect pick-me-up when you need a quick and convenient snack on-the-go. Feel free to customize them with your favorite add-ins like dried fruit, coconut flakes, or seeds to suit your taste preferences.

86. Blueberry crisp with oat crumble topping

Ingredients:
For the blueberry filling:
- 4 cups fresh or frozen blueberries
- 1/4 cup granulated sugar
- 1 tablespoon lemon juice
- 1 tablespoon cornstarch

For the oat crumble topping:
- 1 cup old-fashioned rolled oats
- 1/2 cup all-purpose flour
- 1/2 cup brown sugar (packed)
- 1/2 teaspoon ground cinnamon
- 1/4 teaspoon salt
- 1/2 cup unsalted butter, cold and cut into small cubes

Instructions:
1. Preheat your oven to 350°F (175°C).
Grease a 9x9-inch baking dish or similar-sized dish with butter or non-stick cooking spray.

2. In a large mixing bowl, combine the blueberries, granulated sugar, lemon juice, and cornstarch. Stir gently until the blueberries are evenly coated with the sugar mixture.

3. Pour the blueberry mixture into the prepared baking dish and spread it out into an even layer.

4. In a separate mixing bowl, combine the old-fashioned rolled oats, all-purpose flour, brown sugar, ground cinnamon, and salt. Mix well to combine.

5. Add the cold, cubed unsalted butter to the oat mixture. Using a pastry cutter or your fingers, work the butter into the dry ingredients until the mixture resembles coarse crumbs. Some larger chunks of butter are okay and will create a more textured topping.

6. Sprinkle the oat crumble topping evenly over the blueberry filling in the baking dish.

7. Place the baking dish in the preheated oven and bake for 35-40 minutes, or until the blueberry filling is bubbly and the oat crumble topping is golden brown and crispy.

8. Once done, remove the blueberry crisp from the oven and let it cool slightly before serving.

9. Serve the blueberry crisp warm, either on its own or with a scoop of vanilla ice cream or a dollop of whipped cream.

10. Enjoy your homemade blueberry crisp with oat crumble topping as a delicious and comforting dessert!

This dessert is best enjoyed fresh from the oven, but any leftovers can be stored in an airtight container in the refrigerator for up to 3 days. Simply reheat individual servings in the microwave before serving again.

87. Figs stuffed with goat cheese and honey

Ingredients:
1. Chicken breasts
2. Balsamic glaze
3. Olive oil
4. Garlic (minced)
5. Fresh rosemary (or dried rosemary)

Instructions:
1. Preheat your oven to 400°F (200°C).

2. In a small bowl, mix together the balsamic glaze, olive oil, minced garlic, and chopped rosemary.

3. Place the chicken breasts in a baking dish or on a baking sheet lined with parchment paper.

4. Pour the balsamic glaze mixture over the chicken breasts, ensuring they are evenly coated.

5. Bake the chicken in the preheated oven for 20-25 minutes, or until the chicken is cooked through and no longer pink in the center.

6. If desired, baste the chicken with additional glaze halfway through cooking for extra flavor.

7. Once done, remove the chicken from the oven and let it rest for a few minutes before serving.

Enjoy your delicious and flavorful Balsamic Glazed Chicken! This dish is perfect served with roasted vegetables, salad, or rice. Feel free to customize it by adding additional herbs or spices according to your taste preferences.

88. Yogurt parfaits with berries and granola

Ingredients:
- Greek yogurt (plain or flavored, whichever you prefer)
- Fresh berries (such as strawberries, blueberries, raspberries, or blackberries)
- Granola
- Optional: honey or maple syrup for drizzling

Instructions:
1. In a serving glass or bowl, spoon a layer of Greek yogurt into the bottom.

2. Wash the fresh berries under cold water and pat them dry with a paper towel. Slice any larger berries into smaller pieces if desired.

3. Add a layer of fresh berries on top of the Greek yogurt.

4. Sprinkle a layer of granola over the berries.

5. Repeat the layers until the glass or bowl is filled, ending with a layer of granola on top.

6. Optional: Drizzle a small amount of honey or maple syrup over the top of the parfait for added sweetness, if desired.

7. Serve the yogurt parfaits with berries and granola immediately and enjoy them as a nutritious and delicious breakfast or snack option!

These yogurt parfaits are customizable and versatile, so feel free to experiment with different combinations of fruits, yogurt flavors, and granola varieties to suit your taste preferences. They're perfect for meal prep and can be assembled in advance for a quick and convenient grab-and-go option.

89. Whole wheat carrot cake muffins

Ingredients:
- 1 1/2 cups whole wheat flour
- 1 teaspoon baking powder
- 1/2 teaspoon baking soda
- 1/2 teaspoon ground cinnamon
- 1/4 teaspoon ground nutmeg
- 1/4 teaspoon salt
- 1/2 cup unsweetened applesauce
- 1/4 cup honey or maple syrup
- 1/4 cup olive oil or melted coconut oil
- 2 large eggs
- 1 teaspoon vanilla extract
- 1 1/2 cups grated carrots (about 2-3 medium carrots)
- 1/4 cup chopped walnuts or pecans (optional)
- 1/4 cup raisins or dried cranberries (optional)

Instructions:

1. Preheat your oven to 350°F (175°C). Grease or line a muffin tin with paper liners.

2. In a large mixing bowl, whisk together the whole wheat flour, baking powder, baking soda, ground cinnamon, ground nutmeg, and salt until well combined.

3. In a separate mixing bowl, combine the unsweetened applesauce, honey or maple syrup, olive oil or melted coconut oil, eggs, and vanilla extract. Whisk until smooth and well combined.

4. Pour the wet ingredients into the dry ingredients and stir until just combined. Be careful not to overmix.

5. Fold in the grated carrots, chopped nuts (if using), and raisins or dried cranberries (if using) until evenly distributed throughout the batter.

6. Divide the batter evenly among the prepared muffin cups, filling each cup about 3/4 full.

7. Optional: sprinkle additional chopped nuts or a sprinkle of cinnamon on top of each muffin for decoration.

8. Bake the muffins in the preheated oven for 18-20 minutes, or until a toothpick inserted into the center comes out clean.

9. Once done, remove the muffins from the oven and let them cool in the muffin tin for a few minutes before transferring them to a wire rack to cool completely.

10. Serve the whole wheat carrot cake muffins warm or at room temperature. Enjoy them as a wholesome breakfast or snack option!

These muffins are moist, flavorful, and packed with nutrients from the whole wheat flour and grated carrots. They're a perfect way to satisfy your sweet tooth while still enjoying a nutritious treat. Feel free to customize them with your favorite mix-ins like shredded coconut or chopped pineapple for extra flavor!

90. Coconut chia seed pudding

Ingredients:
- 1/4 cup chia seeds
- 1 cup coconut milk (canned or homemade)
- 1 tablespoon maple syrup or honey (adjust to taste)
- 1/2 teaspoon vanilla extract
- Optional toppings: shredded coconut, fresh berries, sliced mango, chopped nuts

Instructions:
1. In a mixing bowl or jar, combine the chia seeds, coconut milk, maple syrup or honey, and vanilla extract.

2. Stir the ingredients together until well combined.

3. Cover the bowl or jar and refrigerate the coconut chia seed pudding mixture for at least 4 hours or overnight to allow the chia seeds to absorb the liquid and thicken the pudding.

4. After chilling, give the pudding a good stir to redistribute the chia seeds evenly throughout the mixture. If the pudding is too thick, you can add a splash of coconut milk to reach your desired consistency.

5. Taste the pudding and adjust the sweetness if necessary by adding more maple syrup or honey.

6. Once the coconut chia seed pudding is ready, divide it into serving bowls or glasses.

7. Optional: Top the pudding with shredded coconut, fresh berries, sliced mango, chopped nuts, or any other desired toppings.

8. Serve the coconut chia seed pudding chilled and enjoy it as a delicious and nutritious dessert or snack!

This pudding is rich in fiber, omega-3 fatty acids, and antioxidants from the chia seeds and coconut milk. It's a perfect make-ahead option for a quick and healthy breakfast or a satisfying dessert. Feel free to customize it with your favorite toppings and flavorings to suit your taste preferences!

91. Creamy Chicken Alfredo Pasta (strained)

Ingredients:
- 8 ounces fettuccine pasta (or any pasta of your choice)
- 2 boneless, skinless chicken breasts, cut into bite-sized pieces
- Salt and pepper, to taste
- 2 tablespoons olive oil
- 2 cloves garlic, minced
- 1 cup heavy cream
- 1/2 cup grated Parmesan cheese
- 2 tablespoons unsalted butter
- Fresh parsley, chopped (for garnish, optional)

Instructions:
1. Cook the pasta according to the package instructions until al dente. Drain and set aside.

2. Season the chicken breast pieces with salt and pepper to taste.

3. In a large skillet, heat the olive oil over medium-high heat. Add the seasoned chicken pieces and cook until they are golden brown and cooked through, about 5-7 minutes per side. Remove the chicken from the skillet and set aside.

4. In the same skillet, add the minced garlic and cook for 1-2 minutes, or until fragrant.

5. Reduce the heat to medium-low and pour in the heavy cream. Stir well to combine with the garlic, scraping up any browned bits from the bottom of the skillet.

6. Add the grated Parmesan cheese to the skillet and stir until the cheese has melted and the sauce is smooth and creamy.

7. Return the cooked chicken to the skillet and toss to coat it evenly with the Alfredo sauce.

8. Add the cooked pasta to the skillet and toss until it is well coated with the sauce.

9. Cook for an additional 2-3 minutes, or until the pasta is heated through and the sauce has thickened slightly.

10. Remove the skillet from the heat and stir in the unsalted butter until melted and incorporated into the sauce.

11. Garnish the creamy chicken Alfredo pasta with chopped fresh parsley, if desired, and serve immediately.

92. Cheese Ravioli in Cream Sauce

Ingredients:
- 1 pound cheese ravioli (fresh or frozen)
- 2 tablespoons unsalted butter
- 2 cloves garlic, minced
- 1 cup heavy cream
- 1/2 cup grated Parmesan cheese, plus more for serving
- Salt and pepper, to taste
- Fresh parsley, chopped (for garnish, optional)

Instructions:
1. Cook the cheese ravioli according to the package instructions until al dente. Drain and set aside, reserving some pasta water.

2. In a large skillet, melt the unsalted butter over medium heat. Add the minced garlic and cook for 1-2 minutes, or until fragrant.

3. Pour in the heavy cream and stir well to combine with the garlic and butter.

4. Bring the cream sauce to a gentle simmer and let it cook for 2-3 minutes, stirring occasionally.

5. Gradually add the grated Parmesan cheese to the skillet, stirring constantly until the cheese has melted and the sauce is smooth and creamy.

6. Season the cream sauce with salt and pepper to taste. If the sauce is too thick, you can thin it out with a little reserved pasta water.

7. Add the cooked cheese ravioli to the skillet and toss gently to coat them evenly with the cream sauce.

8. Cook for an additional 1-2 minutes, or until the ravioli are heated through and the sauce has thickened slightly.

9. Remove the skillet from the heat and transfer the cheese ravioli in cream sauce to serving plates.

10. Garnish with additional grated Parmesan cheese and chopped fresh parsley, if desired.

Serve the cheese ravioli in cream sauce immediately as a delicious and satisfying meal. Pair it with a side salad or garlic bread for a complete dinner experience. Enjoy!

93. Rice Noodles Stir-Fry with Chicken

Ingredients:
- 8 ounces rice noodles
- 2 boneless, skinless
chicken breasts, thinly sliced
- 2 tablespoons soy sauce
- 1 tablespoon oyster sauce
- 1 tablespoon hoisin sauce
- 1 tablespoon sesame oil
- 2 tablespoons vegetable oil, divided
- 3 cloves garlic, minced
- 1 bell pepper, thinly sliced
- 1 carrot, julienned
- 1 cup broccoli florets
- 2 green onions, chopped
- Salt and pepper, to taste
- Optional toppings: chopped
peanuts, cilantro, lime wedges

Instructions:

1. Cook the rice noodles according to the package instructions until al dente. Drain and set aside.

2. In a bowl, combine the thinly sliced chicken breast with soy sauce, oyster sauce, and hoisin sauce. Allow the chicken to marinate for 15-20 minutes.

3. Heat 1 tablespoon of vegetable oil in a large skillet or wok over medium-high heat. Add the marinated chicken and stir-fry for 5-6 minutes, or until cooked through. Remove the chicken from the skillet and set aside.

4. In the same skillet, add the remaining tablespoon of vegetable oil. Add the minced garlic and cook for 1-2 minutes, or until fragrant.

5. Add the sliced bell pepper, julienned carrot, and broccoli florets to the skillet. Stir-fry for 3-4 minutes, or until the vegetables are tender-crisp.

6. Return the cooked chicken to the skillet. Add the cooked rice noodles and chopped green onions to the skillet. Drizzle with sesame oil.

7. Toss everything together until well combined and heated through. Season with salt and pepper to taste.

8. Remove the skillet from the heat and transfer the rice noodles stir-fry with chicken to serving plates. Garnish with chopped peanuts, cilantro, and lime wedges, if desired.

Serve the rice noodles stir-fry with chicken immediately as a delicious and wholesome meal. Enjoy the vibrant flavors and textures of this tasty dish!

94. Macaroni and Cheese (soft texture)

Ingredients:
- 8 ounces elbow macaroni
- 2 tablespoons unsalted butter
- 2 tablespoons all-purpose flour
- 1/4 teaspoon ground mustard (optional, for flavor)
- Pinch of nutmeg (optional, for flavor)
- Optional toppings: breadcrumbs, additional shredded cheese, chopped fresh herbs
- 2 cups whole milk
- 2 cups shredded cheese (such as sharp cheddar or a combination of cheddar and mozzarella)
- 1/2 teaspoon salt
- 1/4 teaspoon black pepper

Instructions:
1. Cook the elbow macaroni according to the package instructions until al dente. Drain and set aside.

2. In a large saucepan, melt the unsalted butter over medium heat. Once melted, whisk in the all-purpose flour to create a roux. Cook the roux for 1-2 minutes, stirring constantly, until it becomes lightly golden in color and has a nutty aroma.

3. Gradually pour in the whole milk, whisking constantly to prevent lumps from forming. Cook the mixture, stirring frequently, until it thickens and coats the back of a spoon, about 5-7 minutes.

4. Reduce the heat to low and gradually add the shredded cheese to the sauce, stirring until melted and smooth. Continue cooking for an additional 2-3 minutes, or until the cheese sauce is creamy and well combined.

5. Season the cheese sauce with salt, black pepper, ground mustard (if using), and nutmeg (if using), to taste. Stir until the seasonings are evenly distributed throughout the sauce.

6. Add the cooked elbow macaroni to the cheese sauce, stirring until well coated and combined.

7. Cook the macaroni and cheese mixture over low heat for an additional 2-3 minutes, stirring occasionally, to ensure everything is heated through and the sauce has thickened slightly.

8. Remove the saucepan from the heat and let the macaroni and cheese rest for a few minutes to allow the sauce to thicken further.

9. Serve the macaroni and cheese hot, optionally topped with breadcrumbs, additional shredded cheese, or chopped fresh herbs for extra flavor and texture.

95. Risotto with Mushrooms

Ingredients:
- 1 1/2 cups Arborio rice
- 4 cups chicken or vegetable broth
- 2 tablespoons olive oil
- 1 tablespoon unsalted butter
- 1 small onion, finely chopped
- 2 cloves garlic, minced
- 8 ounces mushrooms (such as cremini or button), sliced
- 1/2 cup dry white wine (optional)
- 1/2 cup grated Parmesan cheese
- Salt and pepper, to taste
- Fresh parsley, chopped (for garnish)

Instructions:
1. In a medium saucepan, heat the chicken or vegetable broth over low heat. Keep it warm while you prepare the risotto.

2. In a large skillet or saucepan, heat the olive oil and butter over medium heat. Add the chopped onion and sauté until translucent, about 3-4 minutes.

3. Add the minced garlic to the skillet and cook for an additional 1-2 minutes, or until fragrant.

4. Add the sliced mushrooms to the skillet and cook, stirring occasionally, until they are golden brown and tender, about 5-7 minutes.

5. Add the Arborio rice to the skillet and stir to coat it evenly with the olive oil, butter, onions, garlic, and mushrooms. Cook for 1-2 minutes, or until the rice is lightly toasted.

6. If using, pour in the dry white wine and cook, stirring constantly, until the wine has been absorbed by the rice.

7. Begin adding the warm chicken or vegetable broth to the skillet, one ladleful at a time, stirring constantly and allowing each addition of broth to be absorbed before adding more. Continue this process until the rice is creamy and cooked to al dente, about 18-20 minutes.

8. Stir in the grated Parmesan cheese until it has melted and incorporated into the risotto. Season the risotto with salt and pepper to taste. Remove the skillet from the heat and let the risotto rest for a few minutes. Serve the risotto with mushrooms hot, garnished with chopped fresh parsley

96. Baked Ziti (softened pasta)

Ingredients:
- 1 pound ziti pasta (or penne)
- 1 tablespoon olive oil
- 1 onion, finely chopped
- 2 cloves garlic, minced
- 1 pound ground beef or Italian sausage
- 1 (24-ounce) jar marinara sauce
- 1 cup ricotta cheese
- 1 cup shredded mozzarella cheese
- 1/2 cup grated Parmesan cheese
- Salt and pepper, to taste
- Fresh parsley or basil, chopped (for garnish, optional)

Instructions:

1. Preheat your oven to 375°F (190°C). Grease a 9x13-inch baking dish with cooking spray or olive oil.

2. Cook the ziti pasta according to the package instructions until just slightly undercooked. Drain the pasta and set aside.

3. In a large skillet, heat the olive oil over medium heat. Add the chopped onion and cook until softened, about 3-4 minutes. Add the minced garlic and cook for an additional 1-2 minutes, or until fragrant.

4. Add the ground beef or Italian sausage to the skillet and cook, breaking it apart with a wooden spoon, until browned and cooked through.

5. Stir in the marinara sauce and simmer for 5-7 minutes, allowing the flavors to meld together. Season with salt and pepper to taste.

6. In a large mixing bowl, combine the cooked ziti pasta with the meat sauce mixture. Stir until the pasta is evenly coated.

7. In a separate bowl, mix together the ricotta cheese, shredded mozzarella cheese, and grated Parmesan cheese until well combined.

8. Spread half of the pasta mixture evenly into the prepared baking dish. Top with half of the cheese mixture, spreading it out in an even layer.

9. Repeat the layers with the remaining pasta mixture and cheese mixture.

10. Cover the baking dish with aluminum foil and bake in the preheated oven for 20 minutes.

11. Remove the foil and continue baking for an additional 10-15 minutes, or until the cheese is melted and bubbly.

12. Remove the baked ziti from the oven and let it cool for a few minutes before serving. Garnish with chopped fresh parsley or basil, if desired.

97. Rice Pilaf with Soft Vegetables

Ingredients:
- 1 cup long-grain white rice
- 2 cups chicken or vegetable broth
- 2 tablespoons olive oil or butter
- 1 small onion, finely chopped
- 2 cloves garlic, minced
- 1 carrot, diced
- 1 celery stalk, diced
- 1 bell pepper (any color), diced
- 1/2 cup frozen peas
- Salt and pepper, to taste
- 1 tablespoon chopped fresh parsley (for garnish, optional)

Instructions:

1. Rinse the rice under cold water until the water runs clear. Drain and set aside.

2. In a medium saucepan, heat the olive oil or butter over medium heat. Add the chopped onion and cook until softened, about 3-4 minutes.

3. Add the minced garlic to the saucepan and cook for an additional 1-2 minutes, or until fragrant.

4. Stir in the diced carrot, celery, and bell pepper. Cook, stirring occasionally, until the vegetables are softened, about 5-7 minutes.

5. Add the rinsed rice to the saucepan and cook, stirring frequently, for 1-2 minutes to lightly toast the rice.

6. Pour in the chicken or vegetable broth and bring the mixture to a boil.

7. Reduce the heat to low, cover the saucepan, and simmer for 15-20 minutes, or until the rice is tender and has absorbed all of the liquid.

8. Stir in the frozen peas and cook for an additional 2-3 minutes, or until heated through.

9. Season the rice pilaf with salt and pepper to taste.

10. Remove the saucepan from the heat and let the rice pilaf sit, covered, for a few minutes to allow the flavors to meld together.

11. Fluff the rice pilaf with a fork and transfer it to a serving dish. Garnish with chopped fresh parsley, if desired, and serve hot.

98. Spaghetti Carbonara (lightly sauced)

Ingredients:
- 8 ounces spaghetti
- 4 slices bacon, chopped
- 2 cloves garlic, minced
- 2 large eggs
- 1/2 cup grated Parmesan cheese, plus more for serving
- Salt and black pepper, to taste
- Chopped fresh parsley (for garnish, optional)

Instructions:
1. Cook the spaghetti in a large pot of salted boiling water according to the package instructions until al dente. Reserve about 1/2 cup of pasta water before draining the spaghetti. Drain the spaghetti and set aside.

2. While the spaghetti is cooking, heat a large skillet over medium heat. Add the chopped bacon and cook until crispy, about 5-7 minutes.

3. Add the minced garlic to the skillet with the bacon and cook for an additional 1-2 minutes, or until fragrant. Remove the skillet from the heat and set aside.

4. In a small bowl, whisk together the eggs, grated Parmesan cheese, and a pinch of black pepper until well combined.

5. Return the skillet with the cooked bacon and garlic to low heat. Add the drained spaghetti to the skillet and toss to combine with the bacon and garlic.

6. Remove the skillet from the heat and quickly pour the egg and Parmesan mixture over the hot spaghetti, tossing constantly to coat the spaghetti evenly. The residual heat from the spaghetti will cook the eggs and create a creamy sauce.

7. If the sauce is too thick, gradually add some of the reserved pasta water, a little at a time, until you reach your desired consistency.

8. Season the spaghetti carbonara with salt and additional black pepper to taste.

9. Transfer the spaghetti carbonara to serving plates or a large bowl. Sprinkle with additional grated Parmesan cheese and chopped fresh parsley for garnish, if desired.

10. Serve the spaghetti carbonara immediately, while it's hot and creamy.

99. Turkey and Rice Casserole

Ingredients:
- 1 cup long-grain white rice
- 2 cups chicken broth
- 1 tablespoon olive oil
- 1 small onion, chopped
- 2 cloves garlic, minced
- 1 pound ground turkey
- 1 cup frozen mixed vegetables (such as peas, carrots, and corn)
- 1 teaspoon dried thyme
- 1 teaspoon dried sage
- Salt and pepper, to taste
- 1 cup shredded cheese (such as cheddar or mozzarella)
- Optional topping: breadcrumbs

Instructions:

1. Preheat your oven to 375°F (190°C). Grease a 9x13-inch baking dish with cooking spray or olive oil.

2. In a medium saucepan, combine the rice and chicken broth. Bring to a boil, then reduce the heat to low, cover, and simmer for 15-20 minutes, or until the rice is cooked and the liquid is absorbed. Remove from heat and set aside.

3. In a large skillet, heat the olive oil over medium heat. Add the chopped onion and cook until softened, about 3-4 minutes. Add the minced garlic and cook for an additional 1-2 minutes, or until fragrant.

4. Add the ground turkey to the skillet and cook, breaking it apart with a wooden spoon, until browned and cooked through.

5. Stir in the frozen mixed vegetables, dried thyme, dried sage, salt, and pepper. Cook for another 2-3 minutes, or until the vegetables are heated through.

6. In a large mixing bowl, combine the cooked rice and turkey mixture. Stir until well combined.

7. Transfer the mixture to the prepared baking dish and spread it out evenly.

8. Sprinkle the shredded cheese over the top of the casserole. If desired, sprinkle breadcrumbs over the cheese layer for an extra crunchy topping.

9. Cover the baking dish with aluminum foil and bake in the preheated oven for 20-25 minutes.

10. Remove the foil and bake for an additional 5-10 minutes, or until the cheese is melted and bubbly. Remove the casserole from the oven and let it cool for a few minutes before serving.

100. Vegetable Fried Rice (soft veggies)

Ingredients:
- 2 cups cooked rice (preferably chilled)
- 2 tablespoons vegetable oil
- 2 cloves garlic, minced
- 1 small onion, finely chopped
- 1 carrot, diced
- 1 bell pepper (any color), diced
- 1 cup frozen peas, thawed
- 2 eggs, beaten
- 2 tablespoons soy sauce
- 1 tablespoon oyster sauce (optional)
- Salt and pepper, to taste
- 2 green onions, chopped (for garnish, optional)
- Sesame seeds (for garnish, optional)

Instructions:
1. Heat 1 tablespoon of vegetable oil in a large skillet or wok over medium heat. Add the beaten eggs and scramble until cooked through. Remove the eggs from the skillet and set aside.

2. In the same skillet, add the remaining tablespoon of vegetable oil. Add the minced garlic and chopped onion, and sauté until softened, about 3-4 minutes.

3. Add the diced carrot and bell pepper to the skillet. Cook, stirring occasionally, until the vegetables are tender, about 5-7 minutes.

4. Stir in the thawed peas and cooked rice. Cook, stirring frequently, until the rice is heated through.

5. Push the rice and vegetables to one side of the skillet, and pour the beaten eggs into the empty space. Scramble the eggs until they are fully cooked.

6. Stir the scrambled eggs into the rice and vegetable mixture.

7. Drizzle the soy sauce and oyster sauce (if using) over the fried rice. Season with salt and pepper to taste. Stir well to combine.

8. Cook the fried rice for an additional 2-3 minutes, stirring constantly, to allow the flavors to meld together.

9. Remove the skillet from the heat and transfer the vegetable fried rice to serving plates or a large bowl. Garnish with chopped green onions and sesame seeds, if desired.

101. Vanilla Pudding Cup

Ingredients:
- 2 cups whole milk
- 1/2 cup granulated sugar
- 1/4 cup cornstarch
- 1/4 teaspoon salt
- 2 large egg yolks
- 2 tablespoons unsalted butter
- 2 teaspoons pure vanilla extract

Instructions:
1. In a medium saucepan, combine the milk, sugar, cornstarch, and salt. Whisk until well combined and there are no lumps.

2. Place the saucepan over medium heat and cook, stirring constantly, until the mixture thickens and comes to a gentle boil, about 8-10 minutes.

3. In a small bowl, lightly beat the egg yolks. Gradually whisk in about 1/2 cup of the hot milk mixture to temper the yolks.

4. Pour the tempered yolks back into the saucepan with the rest of the milk mixture, whisking constantly.

5. Continue cooking for another 2-3 minutes until the pudding is thickened.

6. Remove the saucepan from the heat and stir in the butter and vanilla extract until the butter is melted and the vanilla is well incorporated.

7. Pour the pudding into individual serving cups or ramekins.

8. Press a piece of plastic wrap directly onto the surface of each pudding cup to prevent a skin from forming.

9. Refrigerate for at least 2 hours, or until chilled and set.

10. Serve cold and enjoy!

Feel free to customize your vanilla pudding cups by topping them with whipped cream, fresh fruit, or a sprinkle of cinnamon or cocoa powder. Enjoy your creamy, homemade treat!

102. Applesauce Cup

Ingredients:
- 6 medium-sized apples (such as Gala, Fuji, or Honeycrisp), peeled, cored, and chopped
- 1/4 cup water
- 2 tablespoons lemon juice (optional)
- 2-4 tablespoons granulated sugar (adjust to taste)
- 1/2 teaspoon ground cinnamon (optional)

Instructions:
1. In a medium saucepan, combine the chopped apples, water, and lemon juice (if using). Stir to combine.

2. Place the saucepan over medium heat and bring the mixture to a simmer.

3. Reduce the heat to low and cover the saucepan. Let the apples simmer gently for about 15-20 minutes, or until they are very soft and tender.

4. Remove the saucepan from the heat and let the cooked apples cool slightly.

5. Using a potato masher or a fork, mash the cooked apples to your desired consistency. For a smoother applesauce, you can also use a blender or food processor.

6. Stir in the granulated sugar, starting with 2 tablespoons, and adjust to taste. Add more sugar if you prefer a sweeter applesauce.

7. If desired, sprinkle ground cinnamon over the applesauce and stir to combine.

8. Transfer the applesauce into individual serving cups or containers.

9. Allow the applesauce to cool completely before covering and refrigerating.

10. Serve chilled and enjoy your homemade applesauce cups as a healthy snack or dessert!

Feel free to adjust the sweetness and spices according to your preference. You can also experiment with different varieties of apples for unique flavors. Homemade applesauce cups are delicious on their own or paired with yogurt, granola, or even served alongside savory dishes like pork chops.

103. Jell-O Cups (no fruit pieces)

Ingredients:
- 1 (3 oz) package of your favorite flavored gelatin (such as Jell-O)
- 1 cup boiling water
- 1 cup cold water
- Whipped cream or whipped topping (optional), for serving

Instructions:
1. In a heatproof bowl, empty the contents of the flavored gelatin package.

2. Pour 1 cup of boiling water over the gelatin powder. Stir continuously until the gelatin powder is completely dissolved.

3. Once the gelatin powder is dissolved, stir in 1 cup of cold water.

4. Allow the mixture to cool slightly.

5. Pour the gelatin mixture into individual serving cups or molds. Fill them about three-quarters full.

6. Refrigerate the cups for at least 4 hours, or until the gelatin is fully set.

7. Once the gelatin is set, you can optionally top each cup with whipped cream or whipped topping before serving.

8. Serve the Jell-O cups chilled and enjoy their wiggly, colorful goodness!

You can use any flavor of gelatin you like, such as strawberry, cherry, lime, or orange, to make these Jell-O cups. They are perfect for parties, snacks, or desserts and can be enjoyed by both kids and adults alike!

104. Banana Ice Cream (blended bananas)

Ingredients:
- 4 ripe bananas, peeled and sliced into coins
- Optional add-ins:
  - 1/2 teaspoon vanilla extract
  - 2 tablespoons honey or maple syrup
  - 1/4 cup peanut butter or almond butter
  - 1/4 cup cocoa powder
  - A pinch of salt
  - Chocolate chips, chopped nuts, or sliced fruit for topping

Instructions:
1. Place the sliced bananas on a baking sheet lined with parchment paper or a silicone mat. Make sure the banana slices are not touching each other.

2. Freeze the banana slices for at least 2-3 hours, or until they are completely frozen.

3. Once the banana slices are frozen, transfer them to a blender or food processor.

4. If using any optional add-ins, add them to the blender along with the frozen banana slices.

5. Blend the banana slices until smooth and creamy, scraping down the sides of the blender or food processor as needed. This may take a few minutes and may require stopping the blender to push down the banana pieces.

6. Once the mixture is smooth and creamy, transfer the banana ice cream to a freezer-safe container.

7. If desired, fold in any additional toppings or mix-ins.

8. Cover the container and freeze the banana ice cream for another 1-2 hours to firm up.

9. Serve the banana ice cream scooped into bowls or cones, and enjoy your guilt-free frozen treat!

This banana ice cream is naturally sweet and creamy, with endless variations depending on your taste preferences. It's a perfect way to satisfy your ice cream cravings while still keeping it healthy and nutritious.

105. Mashed Berry Compote

Ingredients:
- 2 cups mixed berries (such as strawberries, blueberries, raspberries, blackberries), washed and hulled if necessary
- 2-4 tablespoons granulated sugar, depending on the sweetness of the berries
- 1 tablespoon lemon juice
- 1 teaspoon cornstarch (optional, for thickening)

Instructions:
1. In a medium saucepan, combine the mixed berries, granulated sugar, and lemon juice.

2. Place the saucepan over medium heat and bring the mixture to a simmer, stirring occasionally.

3. Once the berries start to break down and release their juices, use a potato masher or fork to mash them to your desired consistency. Leave some chunks for texture if desired.

4. If you prefer a thicker compote, you can mix cornstarch with a little water to create a slurry and add it to the simmering berries. Stir well to combine and cook for an additional 1-2 minutes until the mixture thickens slightly.

5. Taste the compote and adjust the sweetness if necessary by adding more sugar, stirring until dissolved.

6. Remove the saucepan from the heat and let the compote cool slightly before serving.

7. Transfer the mashed berry compote to a serving bowl or container.

8. Serve the compote warm or chilled, as a topping for pancakes, waffles, oatmeal, yogurt, ice cream, or any other dessert of your choice.

9. Enjoy the burst of fruity flavor in every spoonful of this homemade mashed berry compote!

This compote can be stored in an airtight container in the refrigerator for up to one week. It's a versatile and delicious addition to a variety of dishes and desserts.

106. Rice Pudding with Cinnamon

Ingredients:
- 1/2 cup long-grain white rice
- 4 cups whole milk
- 1/2 cup granulated sugar
- 1/2 teaspoon ground cinnamon
- 1 teaspoon vanilla extract
- Pinch of salt
- Ground cinnamon, for garnish

Instructions:
1. Rinse the rice under cold water until the water runs clear to remove excess starch.

2. In a medium saucepan, combine the rinsed rice and whole milk over medium heat. Bring to a gentle boil, stirring occasionally to prevent sticking.

3. Reduce the heat to low and simmer the rice, uncovered, stirring occasionally, for about 25-30 minutes, or until the rice is tender and the mixture has thickened to a creamy consistency.

4. Stir in the granulated sugar, ground cinnamon, vanilla extract, and a pinch of salt. Continue to simmer for another 5 minutes, stirring occasionally, until the sugar is dissolved and the flavors are well combined.

5. Remove the saucepan from the heat and let the rice pudding cool slightly.

6. Serve the rice pudding warm or chilled, garnished with a sprinkle of ground cinnamon on top.

7. Enjoy the creamy and comforting goodness of homemade rice pudding with cinnamon!

You can also customize your rice pudding by adding raisins, nuts, or a dash of nutmeg for extra flavor. This dessert is best enjoyed fresh but can be stored in the refrigerator for up to 3-4 days. Simply reheat before serving if you prefer it warm.

107. Custard Cups

Ingredients:
- 2 cups whole milk
- 1/2 cup granulated sugar
- 4 large eggs
- 1 tsp vanilla extract
- Pinch of salt
- Ground nutmeg or cinnamon for garnish (optional)

Instructions:
1. Preheat oven to 325°F (160°C).

2. Heat milk until hot but not boiling.

3. Whisk sugar, eggs, vanilla, and salt.

4. Slowly add hot milk to egg mixture.

5. Cook over low heat until slightly thickened.

6. Strain mixture into ramekins.

7. Bake in water bath for 30-35 minutes.

8. Chill for at least 2 hours.

9. Garnish with nutmeg or cinnamon.

10. Serve chilled.

Enjoy the creamy delight of homemade custard cups!

108. Lemon Sorbet

Ingredients:
- 1 cup water
- 1 cup granulated sugar
- 1 cup fresh lemon juice (about 4-6 lemons)
- Zest of 1 lemon (optional)

Instructions:
1. In a saucepan, combine water and sugar. Heat over medium until sugar dissolves completely, stirring occasionally. Once dissolved, remove from heat and let it cool to room temperature.

2. Juice the lemons to obtain 1 cup of fresh lemon juice. Optionally, zest one lemon for added flavor.

3. Mix the lemon juice and cooled sugar syrup together in a bowl. If using lemon zest, add it now.

4. Pour the mixture into a shallow baking dish or metal pan. Cover with plastic wrap and freeze for about 4-6 hours, or until firm.

5. Every hour for the first three hours, remove the pan from the freezer and scrape the mixture with a fork to break up any ice crystals and keep the sorbet smooth.

6. Once fully frozen, scoop the lemon sorbet into serving bowls or cones.

7. Garnish with lemon slices or mint leaves if desired, and enjoy the refreshing citrus taste!

This lemon sorbet is a delightful palate cleanser or a light and tangy dessert. Feel free to adjust the sweetness or tartness by varying the amount of sugar or lemon juice according to your taste preferences.

109. Angel Food Cake (soft texture)

Ingredients:
- 1 cup cake flour
- 1 1/2 cups granulated sugar, divided
- 12 large egg whites, at room temperature
- 1 1/2 teaspoons cream of tartar
- 1/4 teaspoon salt
- 1 1/2 teaspoons vanilla extract
- Optional: Confectioners' sugar for dusting

Instructions:
1. Preheat your oven to 350°F (175°C).

2. Sift cake flour and 3/4 cup granulated sugar together in a bowl. Set aside.

3. In a large mixing bowl, beat egg whites, cream of tartar, and salt on medium speed until soft peaks form.

4. Gradually add the remaining 3/4 cup granulated sugar, about 2 tablespoons at a time, while beating on high speed. Continue beating until stiff, glossy peaks form.

5. Gently fold in vanilla extract using a rubber spatula.

6. Gradually sift the flour mixture over the egg white mixture, about 1/4 cup at a time, gently folding in each addition until just combined. Be careful not to deflate the egg whites.

7. Spoon the batter into an ungreased 10-inch angel food cake pan, spreading evenly.

8. Bake for 35-40 minutes, or until the top is golden brown and springs back when lightly touched.

9. Immediately invert the cake pan onto a cooling rack. Let the cake cool completely in the pan, upside down.

10. Once cooled, run a knife around the edges of the pan to loosen the cake. Carefully remove the cake from the pan.

11. Dust with confectioners' sugar if desired.Slice and serve your soft and airy angel food cake.

110. Soft-Baked Cookies

Ingredients:
- 1/2 cup unsalted butter, softened
- 1/2 cup granulated sugar
- 1/4 cup packed light brown sugar
- 1 large egg
- 1 teaspoon vanilla extract
- 1 1/2 cups all-purpose flour
- 1/2 teaspoon baking soda
- 1/4 teaspoon salt
- 1/2 cup add-ins (such as chocolate chips, chopped nuts, or dried fruit)

Instructions:
1. Preheat your oven to 350°F (175°C). Line a baking sheet with parchment paper or a silicone baking mat.

2. In a large mixing bowl, cream together the softened butter, granulated sugar, and brown sugar until light and fluffy.

3. Beat in the egg and vanilla extract until well combined.

4. In a separate bowl, whisk together the flour, baking soda, and salt.

5. Gradually add the dry ingredients to the wet ingredients, mixing until just combined.

6. Fold in your chosen add-ins (e.g., chocolate chips, nuts) until evenly distributed throughout the dough.

7. Using a cookie scoop or tablespoon, portion the dough into balls and place them onto the prepared baking sheet, leaving some space between each cookie.

8. Bake in the preheated oven for 8-10 minutes, or until the edges are set but the centers are still soft.

9. Remove the cookies from the oven and let them cool on the baking sheet for a few minutes before transferring them to a wire rack to cool completely.

10. Enjoy your homemade soft-baked cookies with a glass of milk or a cup of tea!

These soft-baked cookies are best stored in an airtight container at room temperature and enjoyed within a few days. Feel free to customize them with your favorite add-ins for endless flavor variations!

111. Clear Fruit Juices (strained)

Ingredients:
- Fresh fruits of your choice (e.g., oranges, strawberries, watermelon)
- Sugar or sweetener (optional, to taste)
- Water (optional, for dilution)

Instructions:
1. Wash the fruits thoroughly under cold water to remove any dirt or residue.

2. Peel the fruits if desired, especially for fruits like oranges or pineapples. Remove any seeds or pits.

3. Cut the fruits into small pieces or slices.

4. Place the fruit pieces into a blender or food processor. Add a small amount of water if necessary to help with blending.

5. Blend the fruits until they form a smooth puree.

6. Place a fine-mesh strainer over a bowl or pitcher. Pour the fruit puree through the strainer to remove any pulp or solids.

7. Use a spoon or spatula to press down on the solids in the strainer to extract as much juice as possible.

8. Discard the leftover pulp or save it for other recipes, such as smoothies or fruit sauces.

9. Taste the strained fruit juice and adjust the sweetness by adding sugar or sweetener if desired.

10. Refrigerate the clear fruit juice until chilled, or serve over ice for immediate enjoyment.

You can experiment with different combinations of fruits to create your own unique blends. Clear fruit juices are perfect for staying hydrated on hot days or as a base for cocktails and mocktails. Enjoy the pure, refreshing taste of homemade fruit juice!

As we reach the end of "The Diverticulitis Cookbook: 110+ Delicious and Soothing Recipes," it is our hope that this collection has provided you with not only a wealth of nourishing meals but also a deeper understanding of how to manage diverticulitis through mindful eating. The journey of living with diverticulitis can be challenging, but with the right tools and knowledge, it is entirely possible to lead a fulfilling and healthy life.

Throughout these pages, we've explored a variety of recipes designed to be gentle on your digestive system while still bursting with flavor. From hearty breakfasts that kickstart your day to comforting dinners that bring your evening to a soothing close, each dish has been crafted to support your health and well-being. These recipes are more than just meals; they are part of a holistic approach to managing diverticulitis, emphasizing the importance of nutrition, balance, and enjoyment in your diet.

We have also shared valuable insights into the nature of diverticulitis, helping you understand the importance of dietary choices in preventing flare-ups and maintaining overall digestive health. By following the guidelines and tips provided, you can create a sustainable and enjoyable eating plan that aligns with your health needs.

The recipes and advice in this book are meant to empower you. With practical meal planning strategies, shopping tips, and guidance for dining out, you can confidently navigate your dietary needs in any situation. Remember, managing diverticulitis doesn't mean giving up the joy of eating; it means embracing foods that love you back.

As you continue on your health journey, we encourage you to experiment with these recipes, adapt them to your preferences, and even create your own soothing dishes. Let this cookbook be a foundation for your culinary creativity and a companion in your kitchen.

Thank you for allowing us to be part of your journey towards better health. May the knowledge and recipes shared here bring you comfort, relief, and joy in every bite. Here's to your health, happiness, and the delicious, soothing meals that await you.

Bon appétit and best wishes for a healthy future!